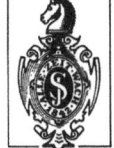

Christine M. Hall · Sundara Lingam

Diagnostic Paediatric Imaging

a case study teaching manual

With 211 Figures

Springer-Verlag
Berlin Heidelberg New York Tokyo

Christine M. Hall, MB, BS, DMRD, FFR, FRCR
Consultant Radiologist, Department of Paediatric Radiology,
The Hospital for Sick Children, Great Ormond Street,
London WC1N 3JH, England

Sundara Lingam, MD(Hons), MRCP, DCH, DRCOG
Consultant Paediatrician, King George Hospital, Eastern Avenue,
Newbury Park, Ilford, Essex IG2 7RL, England

ISBN-13:978-3-540-16202-5   e- ISBN-13:978-1-4471-3125-0
DOI: 10.1007/978-1-4471-3125-0

Phototypesetting by Wilmaset, Birkenhead, Merseyside

2128/3916-543210

Preface

The last decade has seen a rapid expansion in the range and sophistication of diagnostic imaging modalities which are available to clinicians.

Our objective has been to produce a manual on paediatric radiology which will prove of value to those clinicians and radiologists in training who are preparing for the Fellowship, Membership and Diploma examinations of various colleges.

This teaching manual presents radiographs and examples of other imaging modalities from 100 paediatric patients. The material was taken from a radiological teaching collection obtained from patients at The Hospital for Sick Children, Great Ormond Street, over a 10-year period by one of the authors (C.M.H.). With each case a short clinical history is given and a series of questions posed, similar to those encountered in various postgraduate medical examinations. Sample answers with comments and more illustrations are presented on the following page.

It has been impossible to achieve comprehensive coverage of the subject in a book of this size, but we have tried to select examples of those cases which illustrate the range of imaging modalities currently available and which may be encountered both in clinical practice and in examinations.

We acknowledge with gratitude the kind assistance of Miss Sugarhood in the preparation of the manuscript.

London and Ilford   Christine M. Hall
March 1986   Sundara Lingam

Contents

Case 1. **This full-term neonate, now 36 h old, has had progressive abdominal distension since birth.**

Questions:

1. Describe the abnormalities on the supine plain abdominal radiograph (C1.1).
2. What is the cause of these appearances?
3. What is the differential diagnosis?

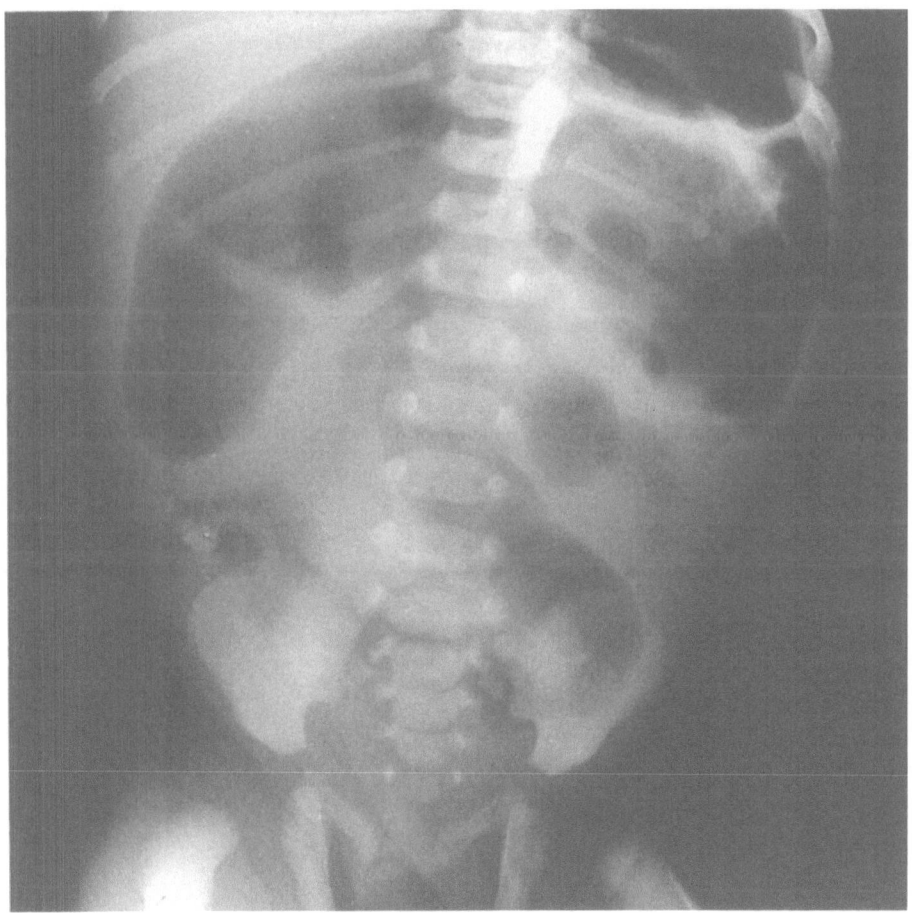

C1.1

Case 1. *Answers:*

1. There are dilated loops of bowel, with no gas in the rectum, indicating obstruction. Calcification is present in the right hypochondrium.
2. Meconium peritonitis as a result of intra-uterine perforation.
3. Causes of low obstruction, which include anorectal atresia, meconium ileus, ileal atresia, Hirschsprung's disease and the small left colon syndrome.

Case 1. *Comments:*

Ileal atresia may occur in a child with meconium ileus and cystic fibrosis secondary to an intra-uterine volvulus of a distended, impacted small-bowel loop. A contrast enema will help to delineate the cause of the low obstruction.

Case 2. This neonate, whose mother was diabetic, presented at 3 days of age with abdominal distension, having passed very little meconium.

Questions:

1. Describe the findings on the supine abdominal radiograph (C2.1).
2. What is the differential diagnosis?
3. What further radiological investigation would you request?

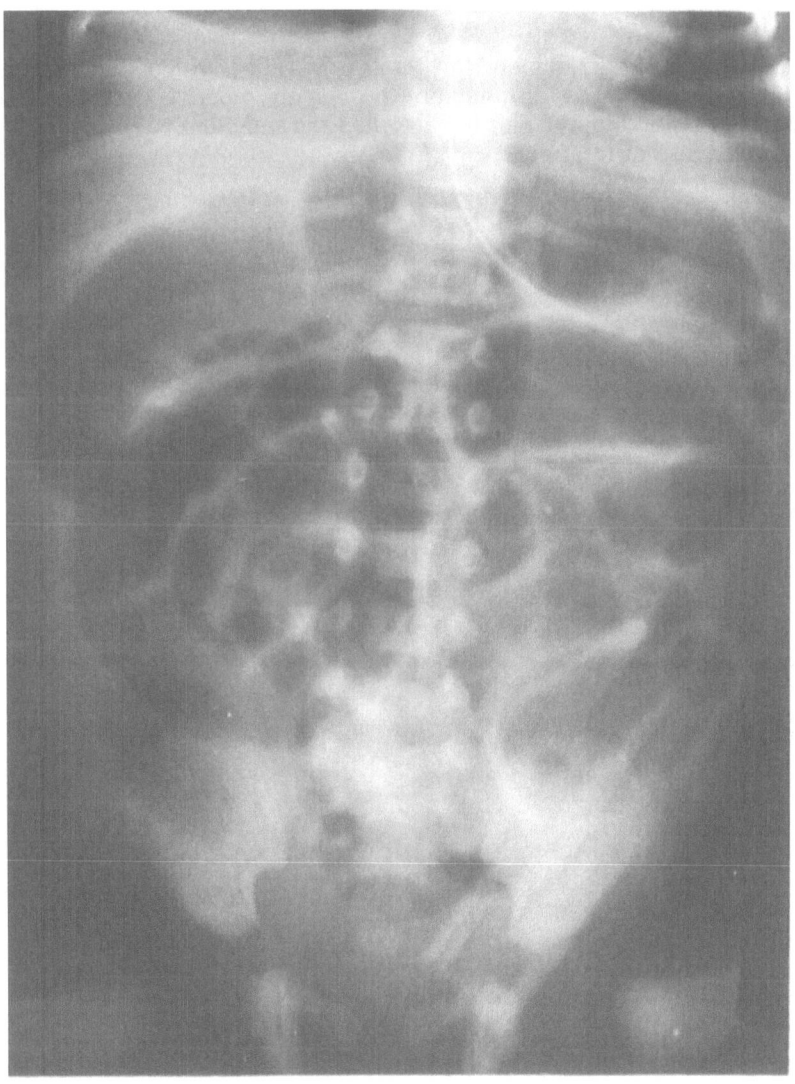

C2.1

Case 2. Answers:

1. Multiple dilated gas-filled loops of gut. At this age differentiation between small- and large-bowel loops should not be made. The large-bowel haustral pattern does not become evident for several months and the diameter of the bowel is also unreliable.
2. Differential diagnosis of a low obstruction includes meconium ileus, anorectal atresia, Hirschsprung's disease, small left colon syndrome and other atresias—ileal and colonic.
3. Barium enema to establish the diagnosis and level of obstruction.

Case 2. Comments:

The contrast enema (C2.2) demonstrates a narrow-calibre colon (microcolon) distal to the splenic flexure with dilatation proximally. Hirschsprung's disease was excluded by rectal biopsy. This neonate had the small left colon syndrome and required no further treatment.

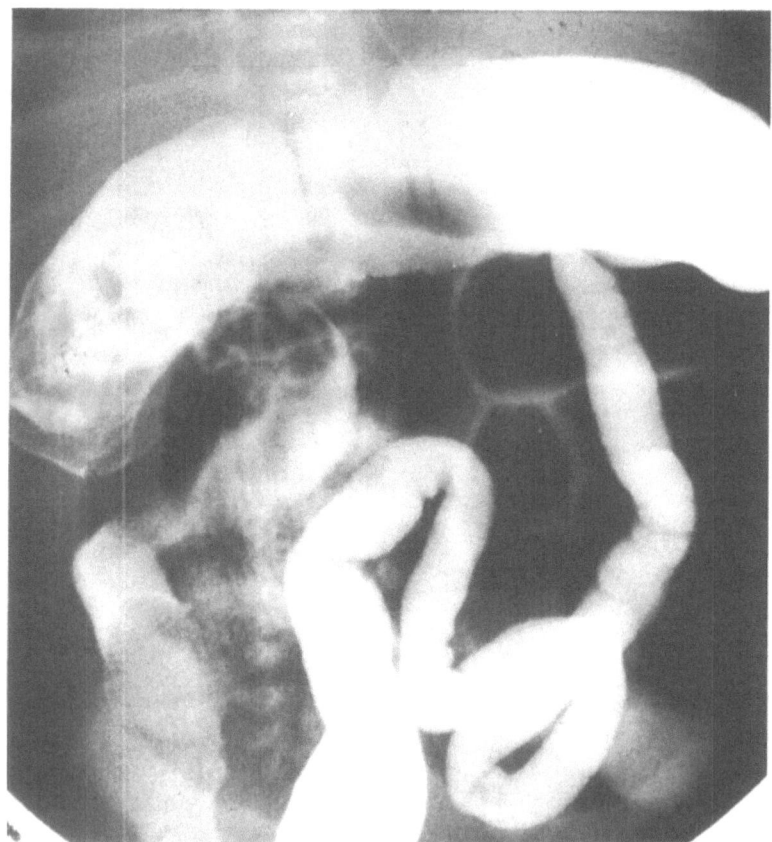

C2.2

Case 3. This 4-month-old infant presented with constipation. There had been delayed passage of meconium in the neonatal period.

Questions:

1. Describe the appearances on this filling film of a barium enema (C3.1).
2. What is the diagnosis?
3. At what stage would you terminate the examination?
4. What contrast medium would you use?

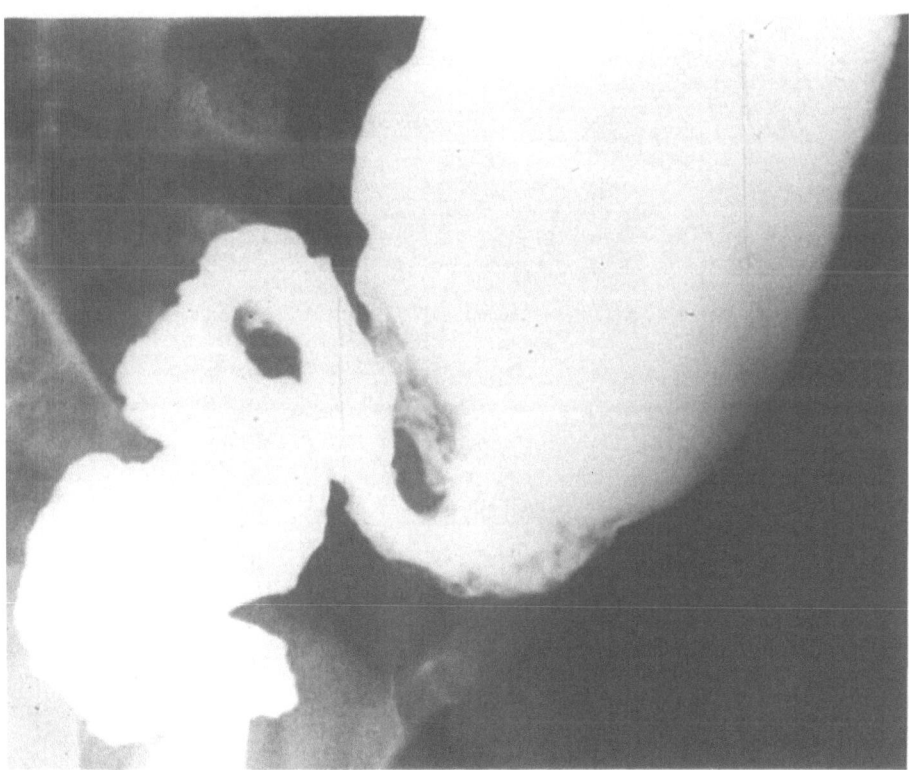

C3.1

Case 3. *Answers:*

1. The rectum and distal sigmoid colon are collapsed with a "serrated" mucosal outline. The proximal sigmoid colon is grossly dilated and there is an inverted cone appearance at the transition zone.

2. Hirschsprung's disease.

3. Once the level of the dilated bowel has been reached or, if the diagnosis is not initially apparent, a delayed 12-h film shows retained barium in the presence of Hirschsprung's disease.

4. Barium, or if excluding Hirschsprung's disease in a neonate with necrotising enterocolitis, a non-ionic water-soluble contrast medium.

Case 3. *Comments:*

The aganglionic zone extends continuously from the anal margin proximally to the normally innervated dilated area of bowel. The zone of transition is normally found in the sigmoid colon. C3.2 is a delayed film on a neonate with long segment Hirschsprung's disease.

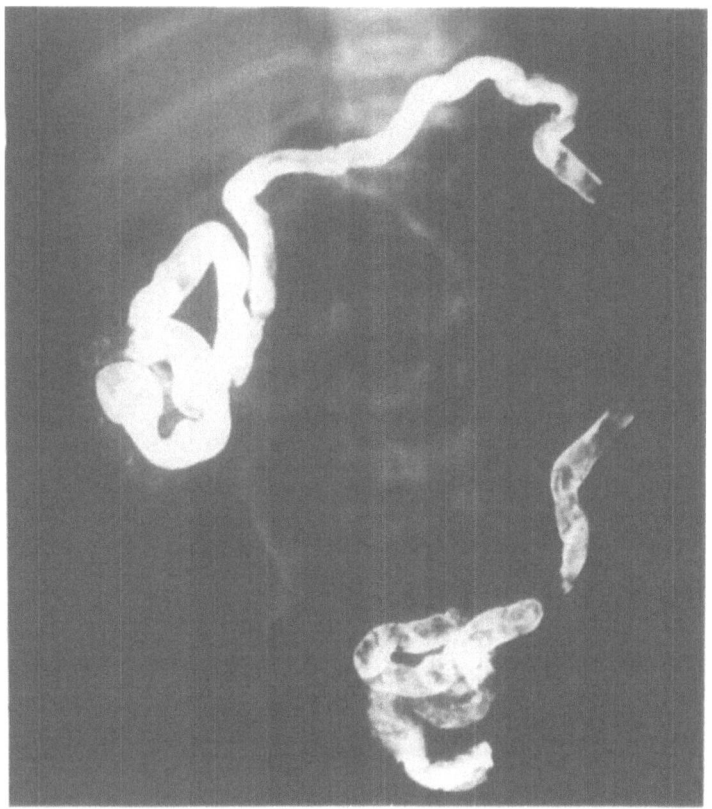

C3.2

Case 4. This 5-day-old term infant had abdominal distension and had passed only a little meconium.

Questions:

1. Describe two significant abnormalities on this erect abdominal radiograph (C4.1).
2. What is the likely diagnosis in this neonate?
3. What would you expect to see on a contrast enema?

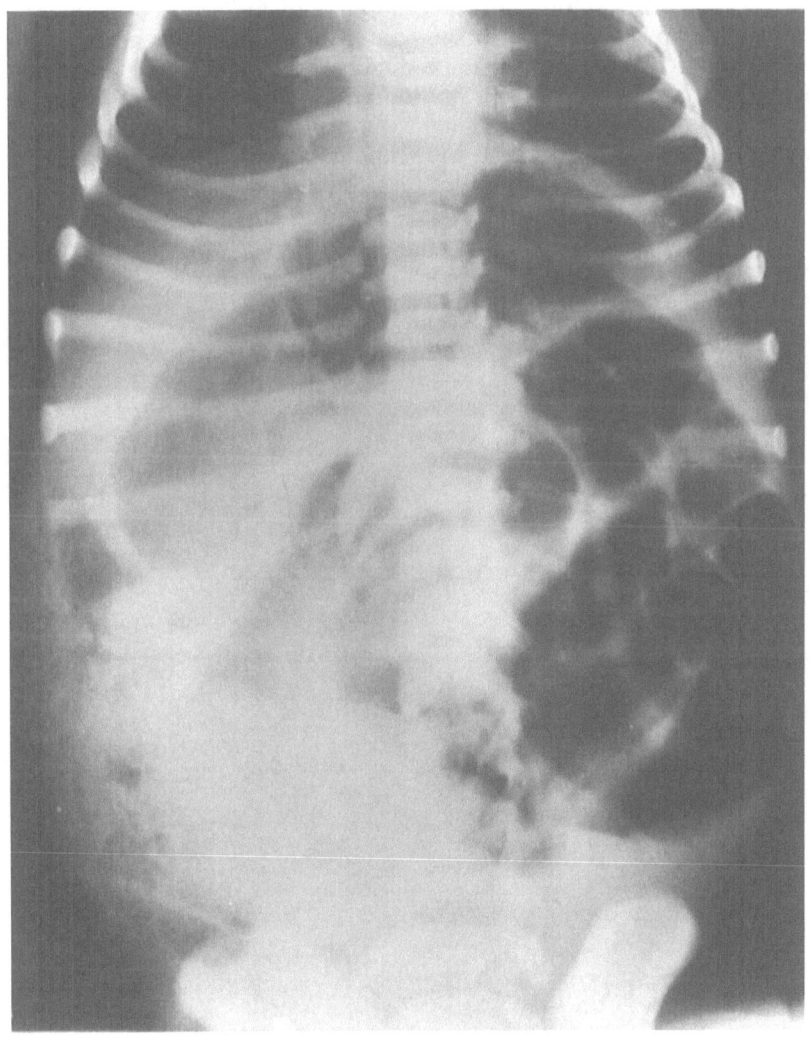

C4.1

Case 4.   Answers:

1. a) Abdominal distension with dilated loops of gut (small-bowel) but without fluid levels.
   b) Granular appearance on the right side due to impacted meconium.
2. Meconium ileus in a neonate with cystic fibrosis.
3. A microcolon, containing a few small pellets of meconium (C4.2).

Case 4.   Comments:

Cystic fibrosis may present in the neonatal period with meconium ileus. Respiratory problems develop later. The absence of fluid levels on the plain abdominal radiograph (C4.1) is characteristic of meconium ileus and is due to increased viscosity. The diagnosis may be established by a barium enema, but a subsequent Gastrografin enema may be curative. Gastrografin is hypotonic, draws fluid into the bowel and contains a "wetting" agent to dislodge sticky meconium from the bowel wall. An intravenous line should maintain correct fluid balance during and after the use of Gastrografin.

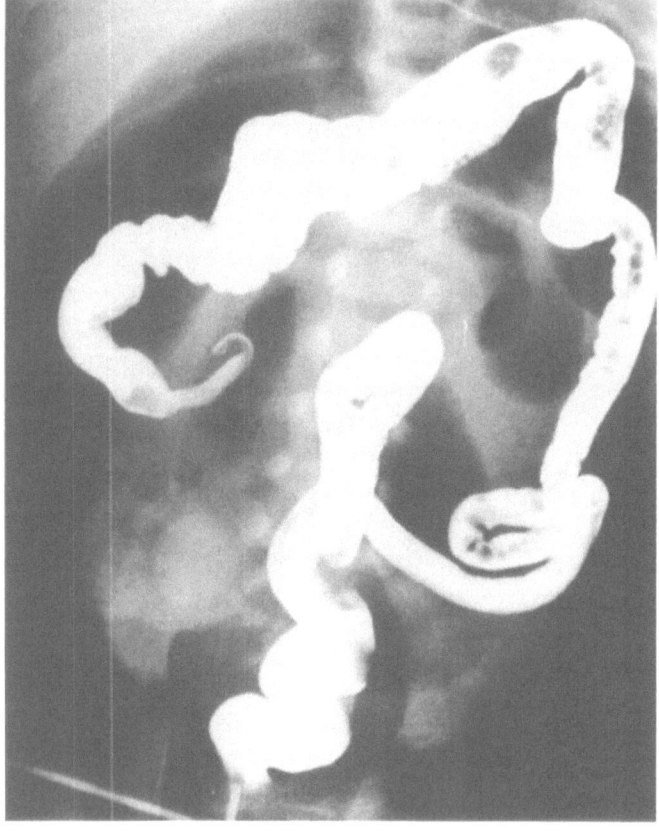

C4.2

Case 5. This term infant was born 24 h previously to a 25-year-old primigravida. She had polyhydramnios and a foetal ultrasound showed distended bowel loops. Two radiographs are shown, one an erect abdomen (C5.1) and the other a prone "shoot-through" lateral abdomen (C5.2).

Questions:

1. Describe two significant abnormalities on these views.
2. What is the diagnosis?

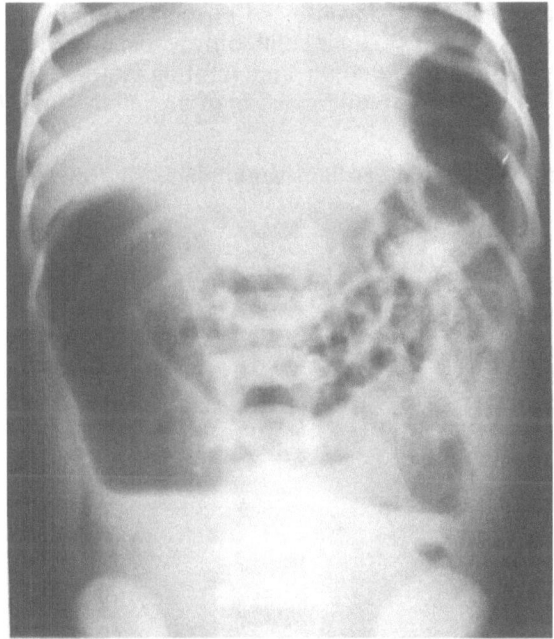

C5.1

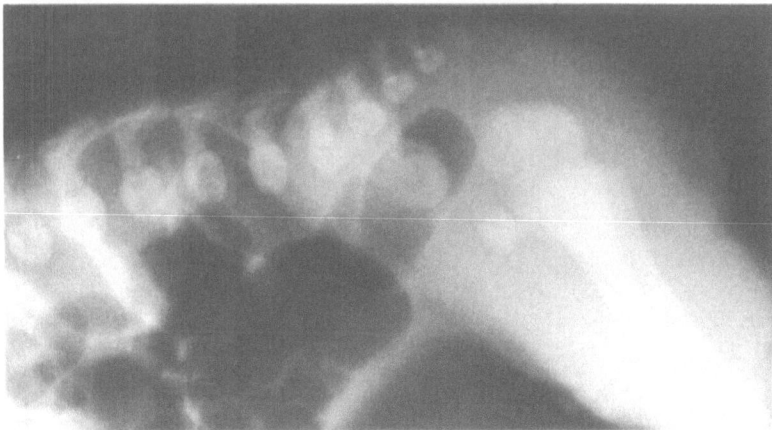

C5.2

Case 5. Answers:

1. a) Multiple dilated loops of gut with fluid levels indicating low intestinal obstruction.
   b) Six lumbar vertebrae.
2. Anorectal atresia (high).

Case 5. Comments:

The prone "shoot-through" lateral view of the abdomen replaces the old "invertogram". In this position, air in the gut rises to the highest point, which is the atretic rectum, and an assessment of the level of the atresia can be made. High rectal atresia (ending above the pelvic floor) is commonly associated with a recto-urethral fistula which may be demonstrated on a micturating cystogram or distal loopogram (C5.3). The VATER association consists of a combination of three or more of:

V, vertebral or vascular—usually congenital cardiac—anomalies, e.g. tetralogy of Fallot

A, anorectal atresia

T, tracheo-

E, oesophageal atresia with or without a fistula

R, renal or radial anomalies.

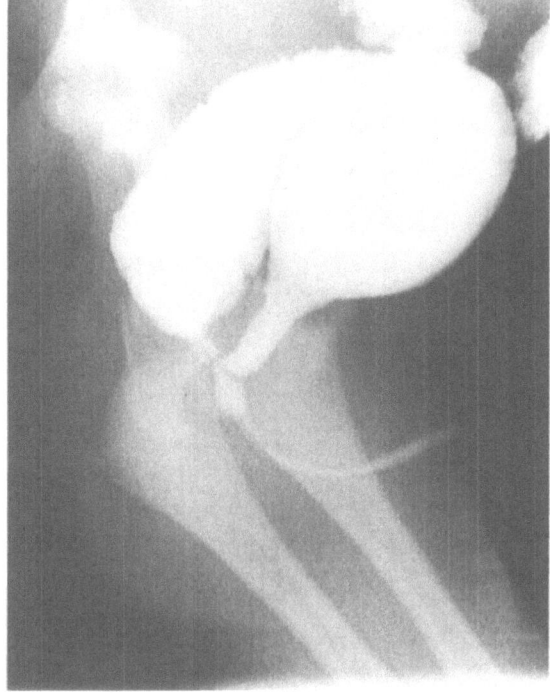

C5.3

Case 6. This abdominal radiograph (C6.1) is of a 2-week-old infant, born at 30 weeks gestation, who had developed marked abdominal distension.

Questions:

1. Describe two significant findings on the radiograph (ignore the circular incubator hole above the gastric air bubble).
2. What is the diagnosis?
3. What other presenting feature would you expect?
4. Name two radiological features indicating a worsening of the condition.

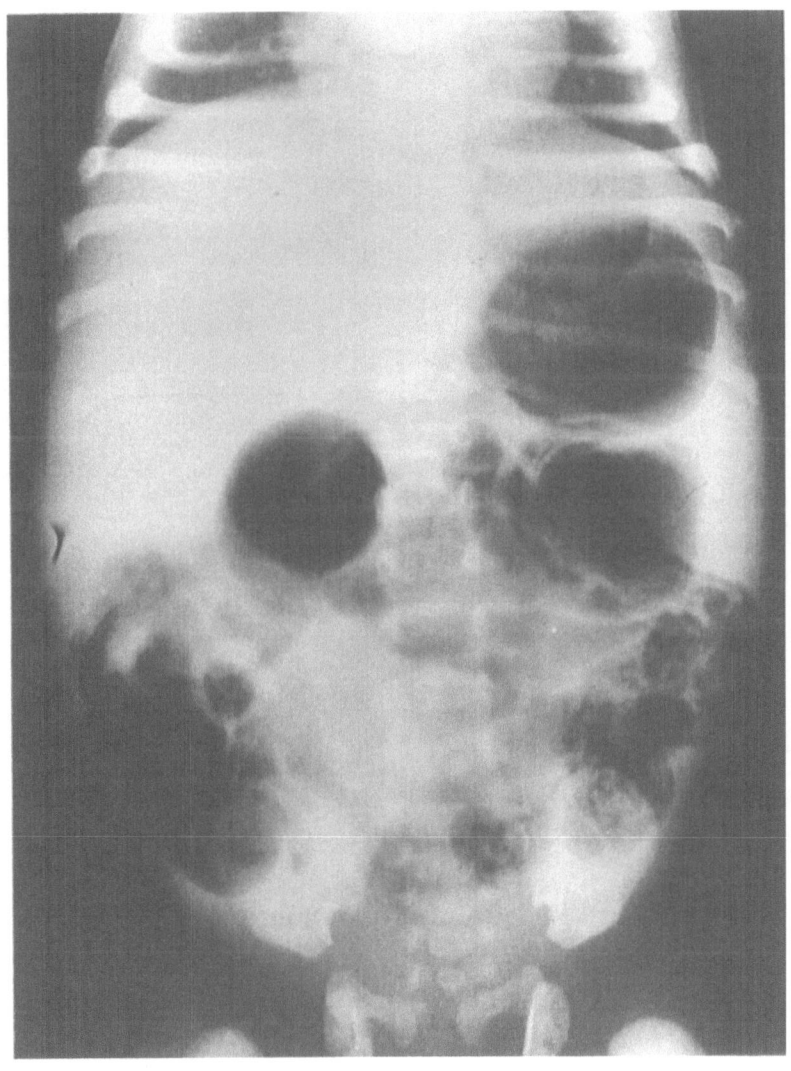

C6.1

Case 6. *Answers:*

1. a) There are dilated loops of gut.
   b) Intramural bowel gas is present on the left side of the abdomen.
2. Necrotising enterocolitis.
3. The passage of blood per rectum.
4. a) Pneumoperitoneum.
   b) Portal vein gas.

The supine abdominal radiograph below (C6.2) demonstrates free air in the peritoneal cavity and scrotum, outlining the liver and the falciform ligament.

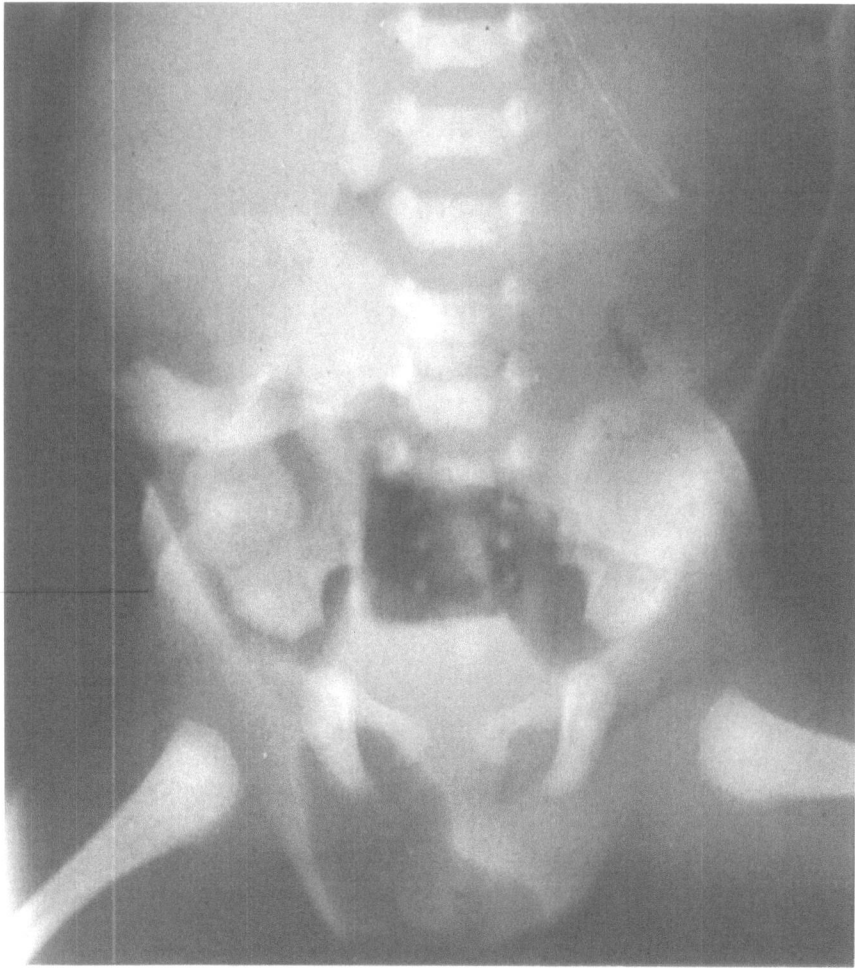

C6.2

Case 7. This neonate presented with abdominal distension and the passage of blood per rectum.

Questions:

1. What abnormality would have been present on the plain abdominal radiographs and what is the diagnosis?
2. Describe the barium enema findings (C7.1).
3. What possible factors predispose to this condition?
4. What are the indications for a contrast enema?
5. What is the contrast medium of choice?

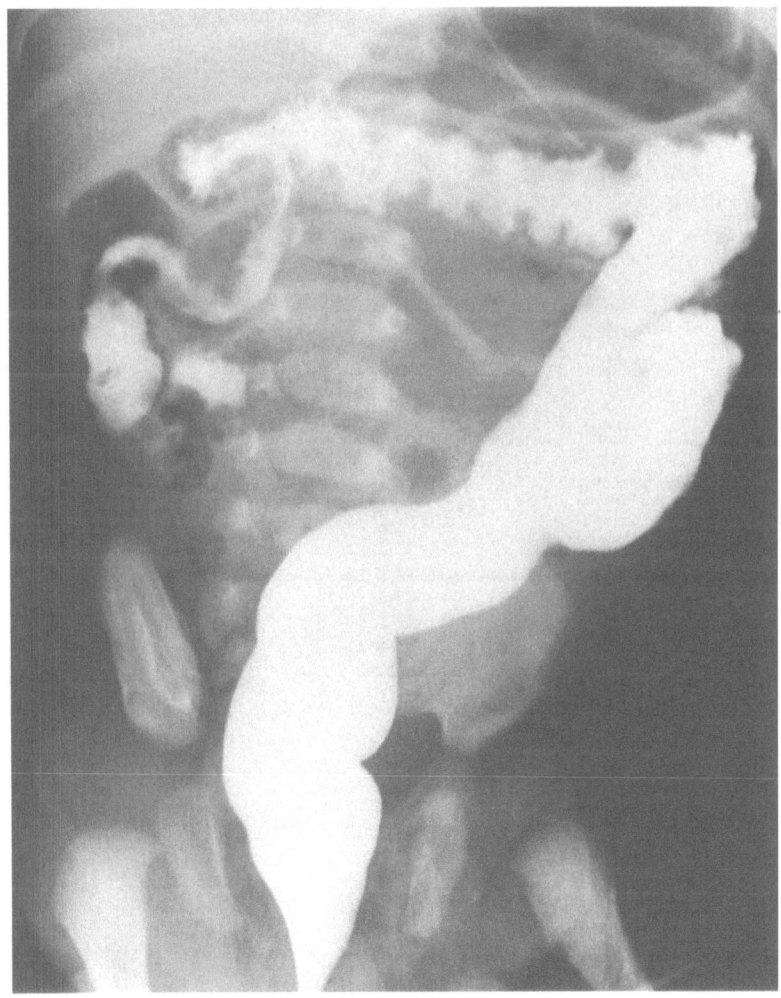

C7.1

Case 7. Answers:

1. Intramural gas with linear radiolucent streaks parallel to the bowel wall.

2. There is gas outlining contrast medium in the ascending and transverse colon. No features of Hirschsprung's disease. The abnormalities are due to necrotising enterocolitis.

3. Prematurity.
   Vascular insults: shock, septicaemia, umbilical catheterisation.
   Mechanical vascular compromise: malrotation.
   Hirschsprung's disease.

4. In the acute phase—in the absence of a recognised predisposing factor and specifically to exclude Hirschsprung's disease.

5. Non-ionic, because of risk of perforation and to prevent electrolyte imbalance.

Case 8. This infant, 4 months of age, presented with vomiting and abdominal distension. She had been treated medically for necrotising enterocolitis as a neonate.

Questions:

1. Describe the findings on this single contrast barium enema (C8.1).

2. What is the diagnosis?

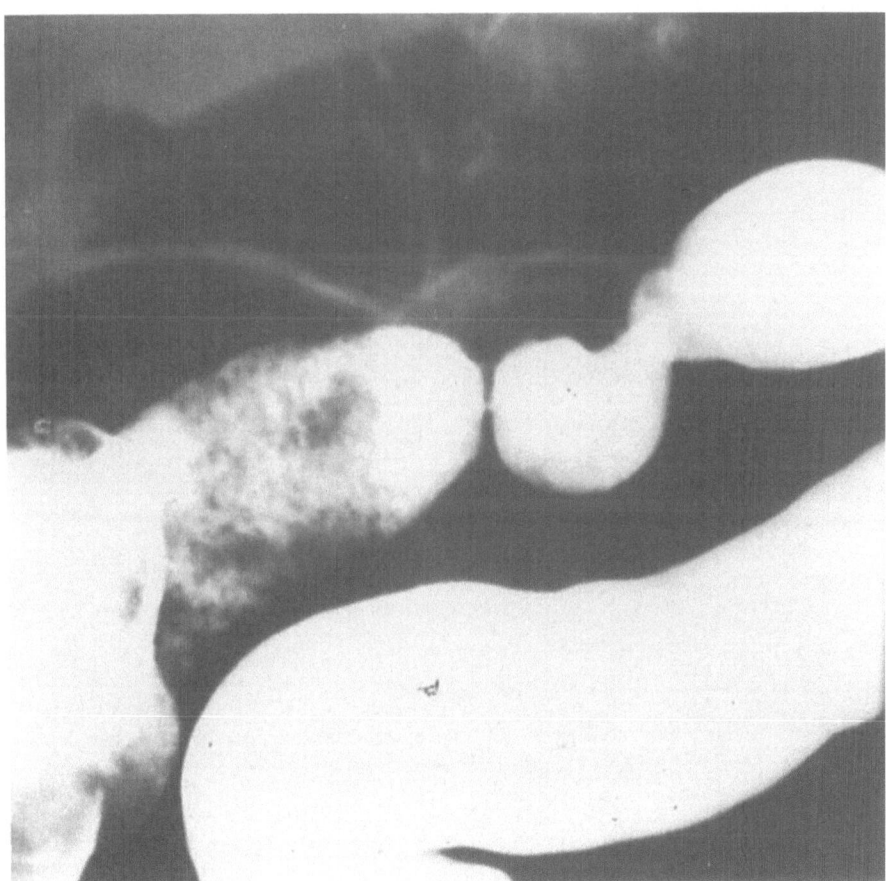

C8.1

15

Case 8. Answers:

1. There are strictures in the mid-transverse colon with faecal retention proximally. Gas-filled, dilated loops of small bowel are present proximally. A nasogastric tube is in position.

2. Colonic strictures following necrotising enterocolitis causing partial obstruction.

Case 9. **The mother of this full-term infant had polyhydramnios throughout pregnancy.**

Questions:

1. What was the clinical presentation?
2. What two abnormalities are present on the radiograph (C9.1)?
3. What is the diagnosis?

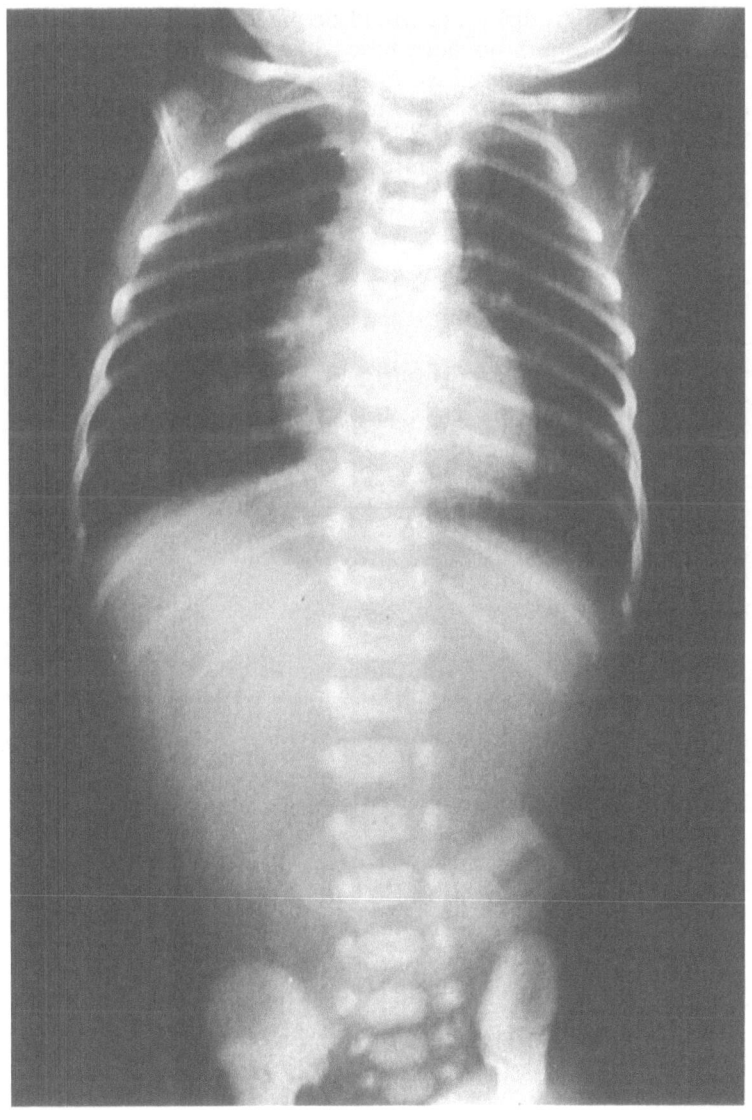

C9.1

Case 9. Answers:

1. Failed passage of nasogastric tube at birth or aspiration of first feed.
2. a) There is a Replogle tube in a blind-ending upper pouch.
   b) No gas is present in the abdomen and there are six lumbar vertebrae.
3. Oesophageal atresia with no distal fistula.

Case 9. Comments:

This type of oesophageal atresia is rare (3% of whole group). If a distal fistula were present (90% of whole group) there would be gas in the abdomen. The Replogle tube is a double-bore radio-opaque tube which is relatively rigid, does not coil in the upper pouch and is used to prevent overspill of saliva into the lungs. At surgery, contrast medium may be introduced into the stomach and refluxed to demonstrate the length of the lower oesophageal segment. The length of the atretic segment determines whether or not a primary anastomosis is possible (C9.2).

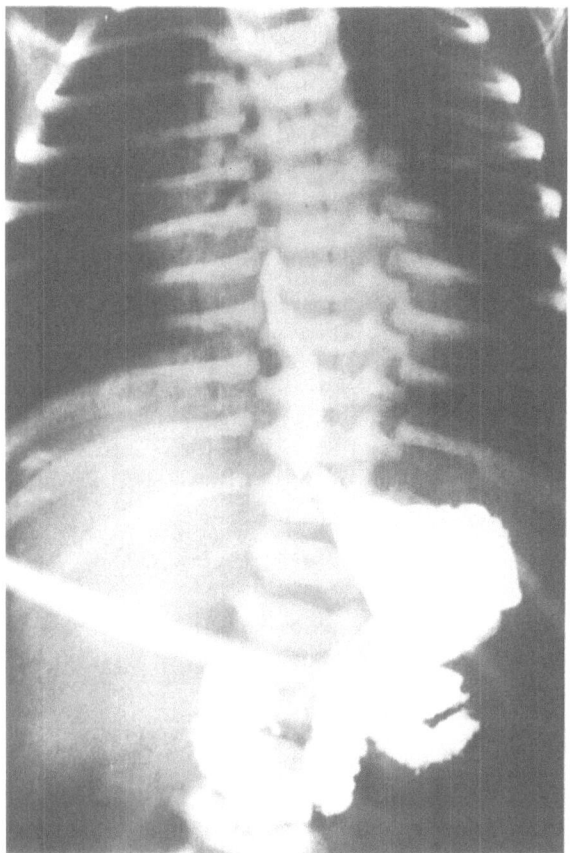

C9.2

Case 10.   This 3-week-old neonate presented with cyanotic spells and coughing during feeds.

Questions:

1. What does this contrast study (C10.1) of the oesophagus demonstrate?
2. Which contrast media are contra-indicated for this examination and why?
3. Why is this study performed with the patient in the prone position?
4. What other congenital anomalies may be associated with this condition?

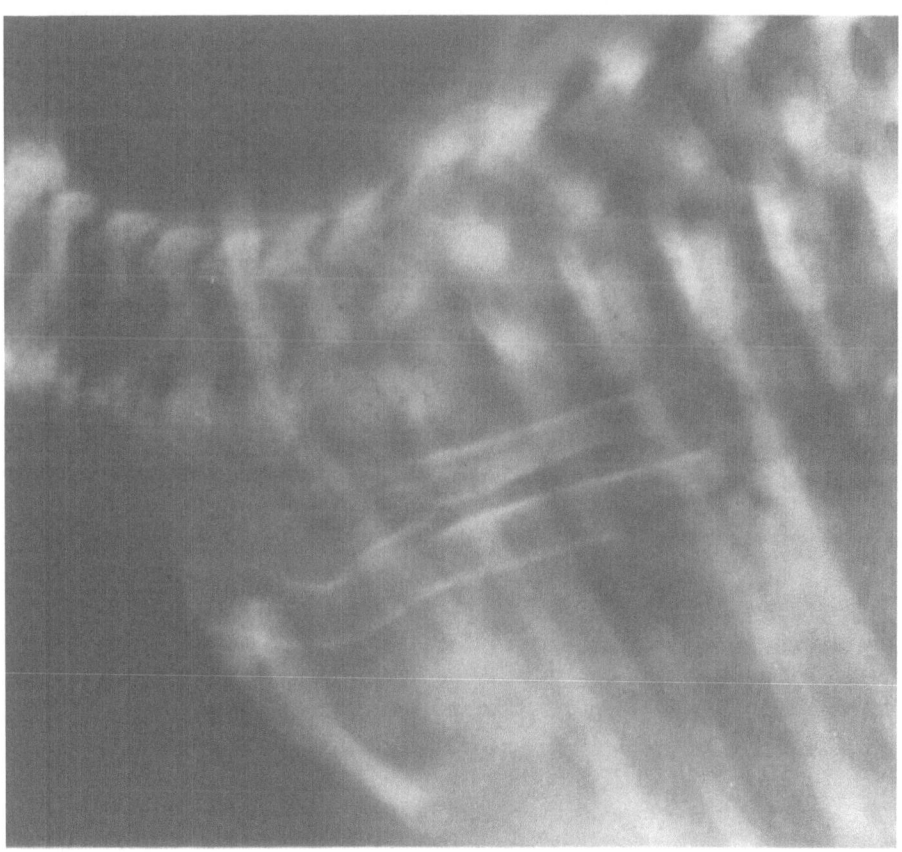

C10.1

Case 10. Answers:

1. An H-type fistula with contrast medium filling the trachea.

2. Ionic water soluble contrast media. If inhaled they may cause an acute pulmonary oedema. The contrast media of choice are non-ionic contrast media and aqueous dionosil. (Barium is an inert substance and may be used under careful screen control to prevent flooding of the bronchial tree).

3. So that gravity may help filling and demonstration of a fistula.

4. VATER association (see p. 10).

Case 11. This 2-year-old child presented with feeding difficulties.

Questions:

1. Describe the abnormal findings on this barium swallow examination (C11.1).
2. What is the differential diagnosis?

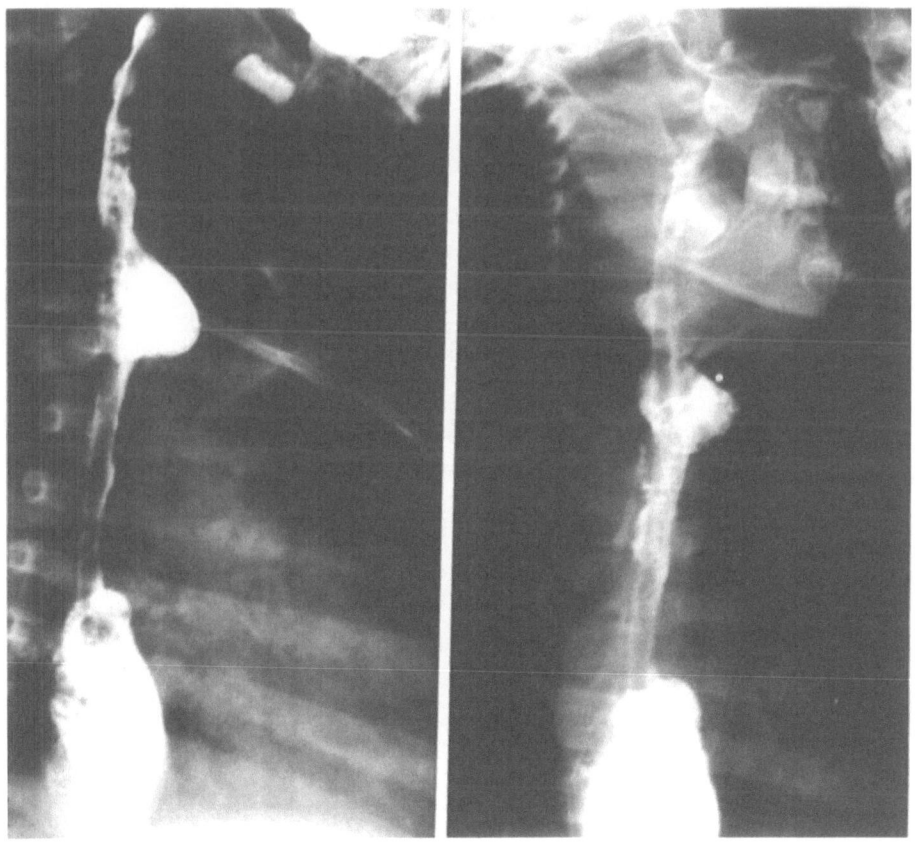

C11.1

Case 11. *Answers:*

1. A nasogastric tube is present. There is a long stricture of the upper and mid oesophagus.
2. Caustic stricture; epidermolysis bullosa. (The abnormality probably extends too high to be a peptic stricture.) This child had ingested caustic soda.

Case 12.   This 8-year-old boy has a sister with identical changes.

Questions:

1. What is the abnormality on this barium swallow (C12.1)?
2. What is the diagnosis?

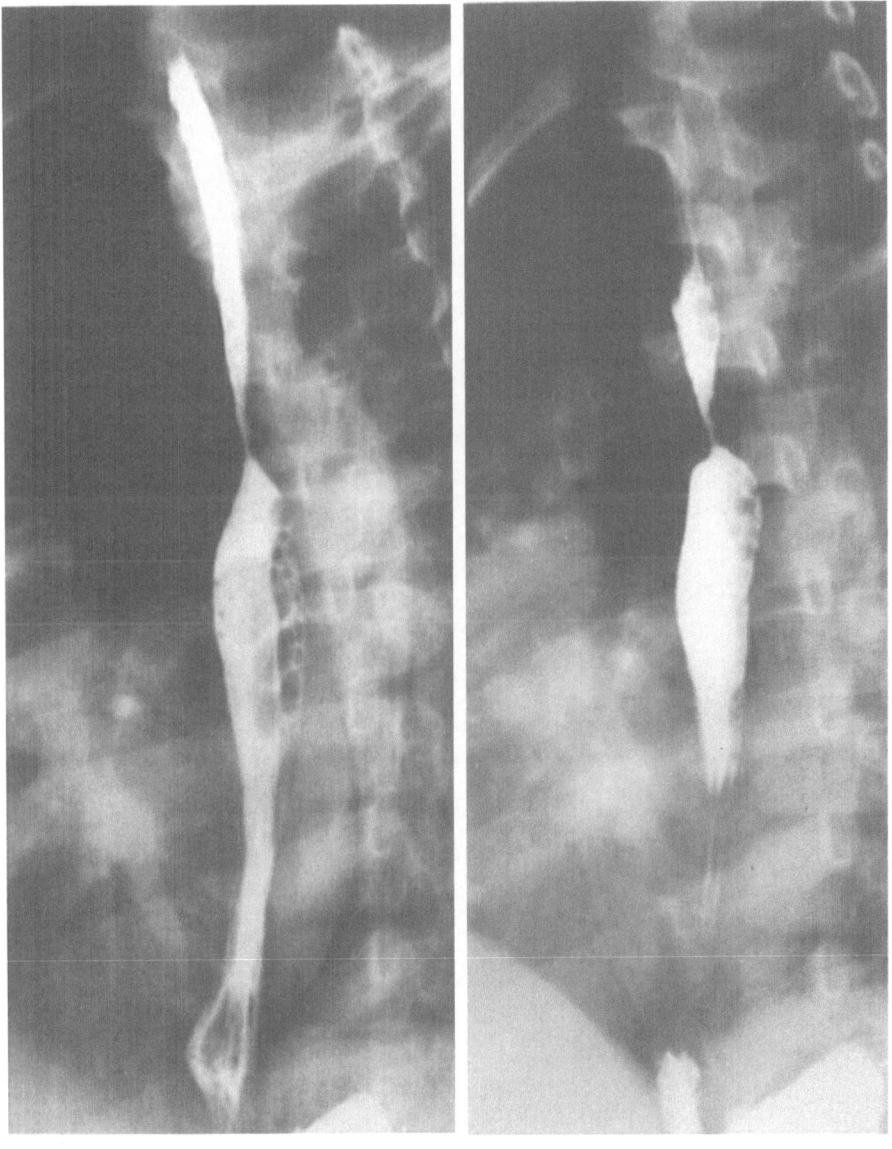

C12.1

Case 12. Answers:

1. A long stricture in the upper-mid oesophagus.

2. Epidermolysis bullosa (ingestion of caustic soda should be considered in a brother and sister).

Case 12. Comments:

Epidermolysis bullosa is inherited in an autosomal recessive manner. The hand changes are illustrated in the severe dystrophic form (C12.2). The bones are slender and porotic. There are fixed flexion deformities associated with soft tissue wasting and contractures. In the milder form of the condition the oesophageal "strictures" are entirely mucosal and resolve rapidly on steroid therapy.

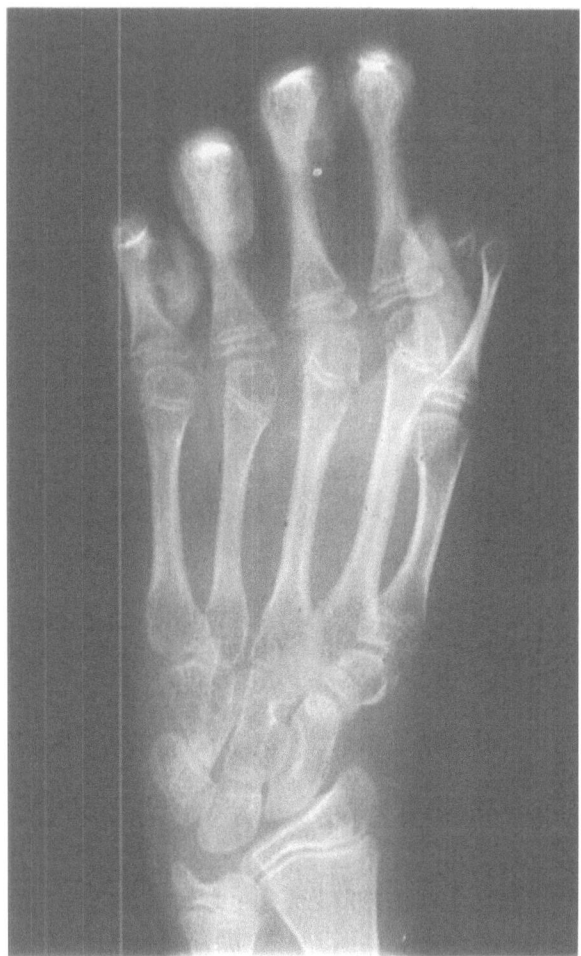

C12.2

Case 13. This 2-year-old child was reluctant to take solid food. The barium meal examination demonstrated marked gastro-oesophageal reflux.

Questions:

1. Describe three other abnormalities on these lateral views of the gastro-oesophageal junction (C13.1).

2. What other abnormalities should be excluded by the barium meal examination?

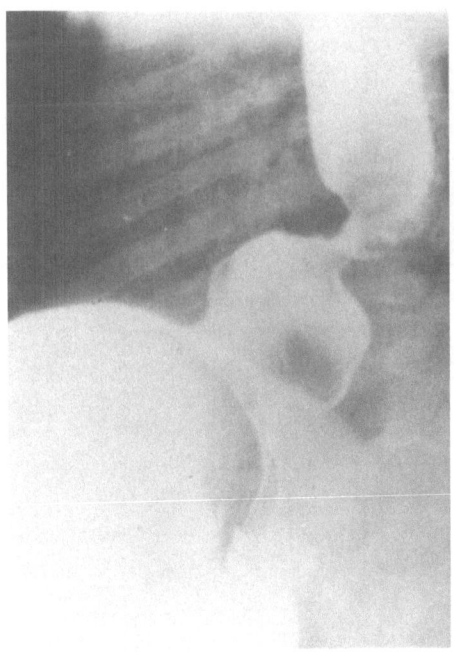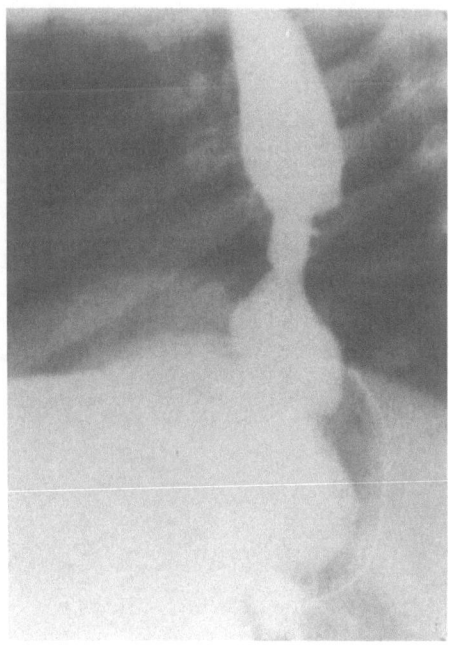

C13.1

Case 13. Answers:

1. a) A sliding hiatus hernia (probably fixed).
    b) A peptic stricture.
    c) Ulceration.
2. A cause for reflux—partial obstruction more distally, usually at the gastric outlet or duodenum, or a higher oesophageal abnormality such as repaired oesophageal atresia (C13.2).

Case 13. Comments:

Peptic strictures are long strictures. Short oesophageal strictures (1–2 mm) may be seen post anastomosis for oesophageal atresia, or may be congenital.

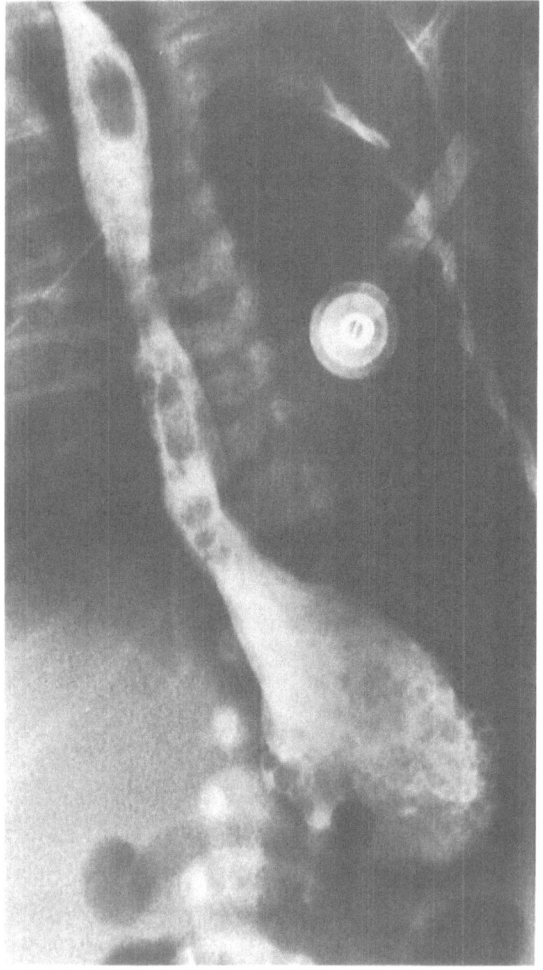

C13.2

Case 14.   This 2-year-old boy with leukaemia refused to eat.

Questions:

1. Describe the abnormality on this barium swallow (C14.1).
2. What is the likely cause?

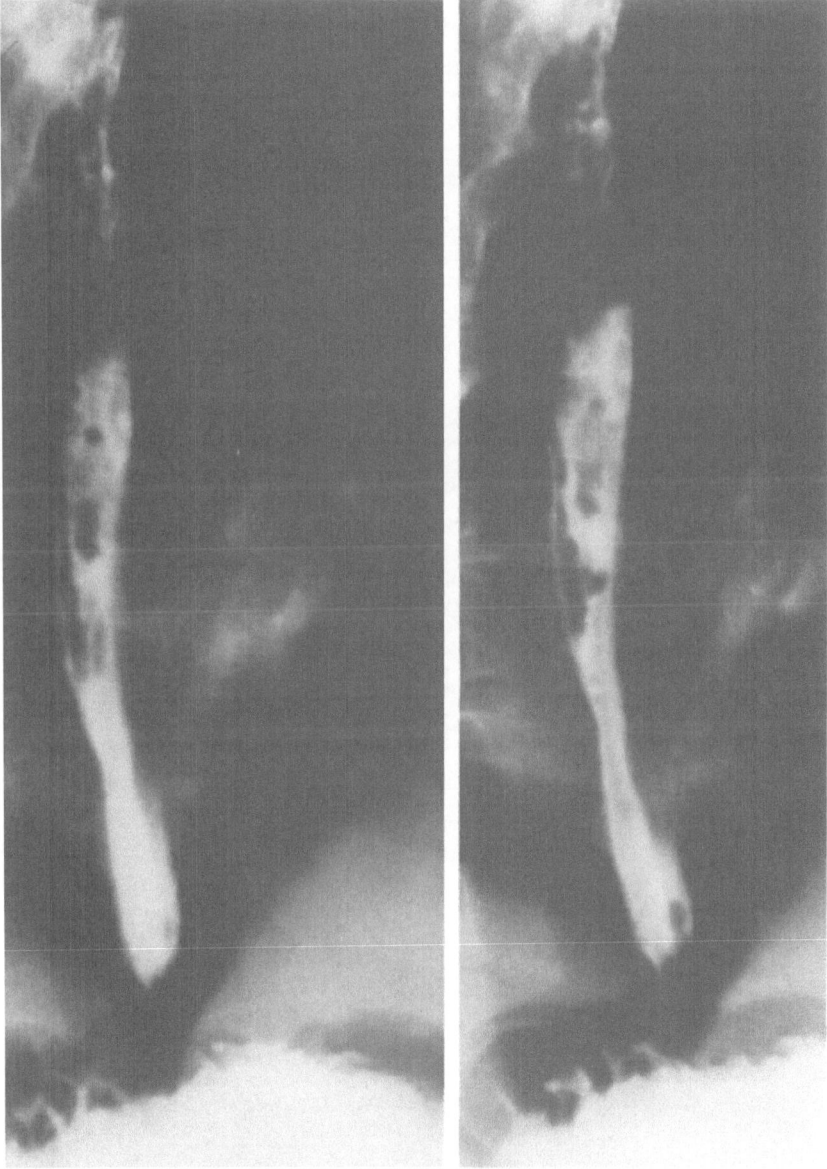

C14.1

Case 14. *Answers:*

1. There are constant linear filling defects mainly in the mid and upper oesophagus.

2. Monilial oesophagitis.

Case 14. *Comments:*

Oesophageal varices in this child with cystic fibrosis (C14.2) may produce a similar appearance but extend upwards from the gastro-oesophageal junction.

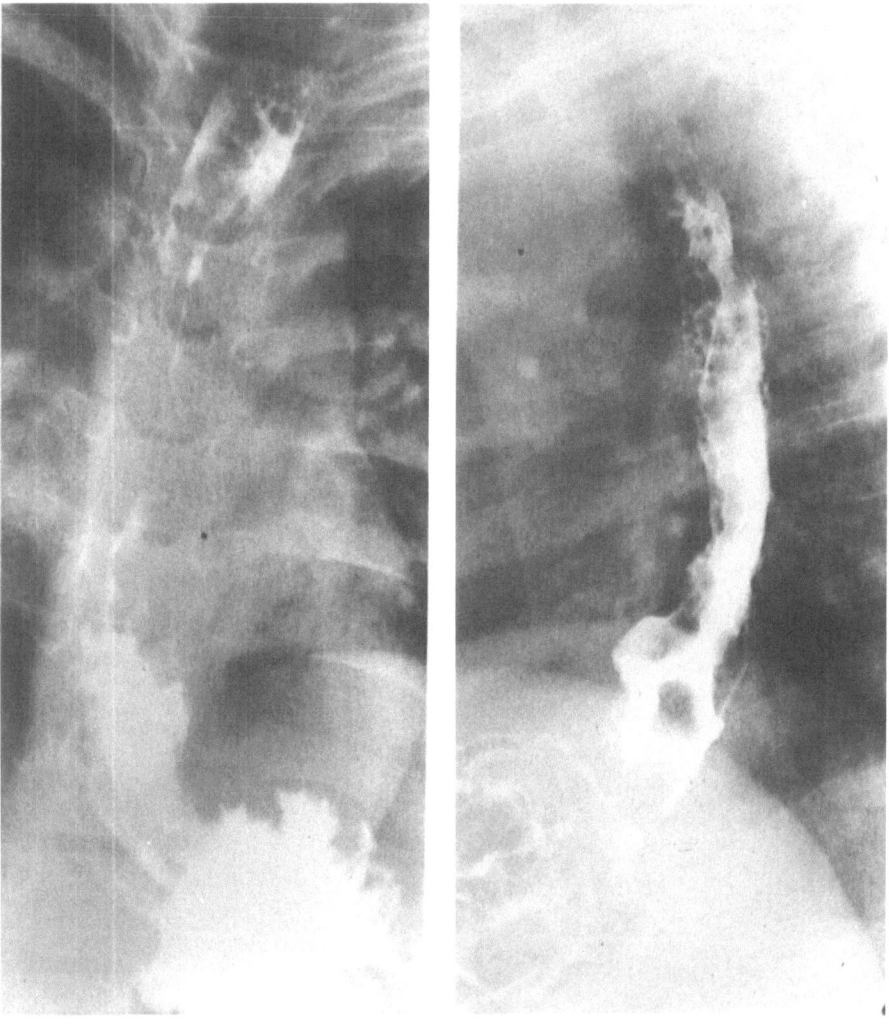

C14.2

Case 15. Plain abdominal radiograph (C15.1) and barium meal film (C15.2) (right lateral oblique view) of a 6-week-old male infant with projectile vomiting.

Questions:

1. Describe two significant abnormalities on the plain abdominal film (ignore the nasogastric tube).
2. Describe the barium meal findings.
3. What is the diagnosis?
4. What other examination would be appropriate?

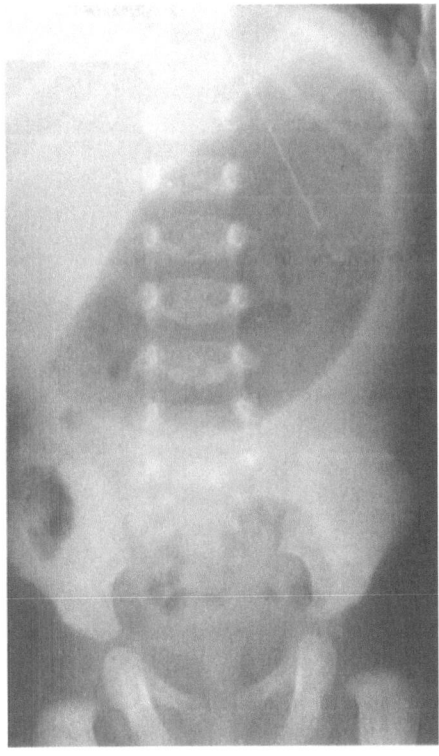

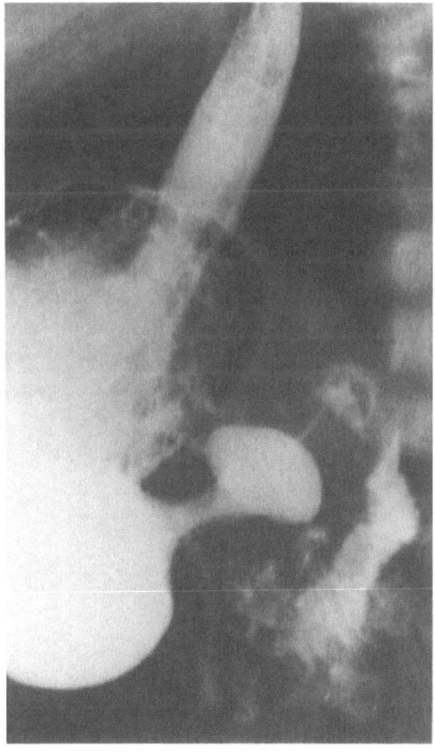

C15.1

C15.2

29

Case 15. *Answers:*

1. a) Gas-filled and distended stomach.
   b) Very little bowel gas distally.

2. There is active peristalsis in the antrum and gastro-oesophageal reflux. A "beak" is present in the long pyloric canal with "shouldering" in the base of the duodenal cap.

3. Pyloric stenosis.

4. Abdominal ultrasound with the stomach distended with fluid to act as a window. If the pyloric muscle measures more than 2 cm (transverse or longitudinal to the pyloric canal) then pyloric stenosis is present. C15.3 is an ultrasound scan transverse to the pyloric canal showing the "target" sign of pyloric stenosis.

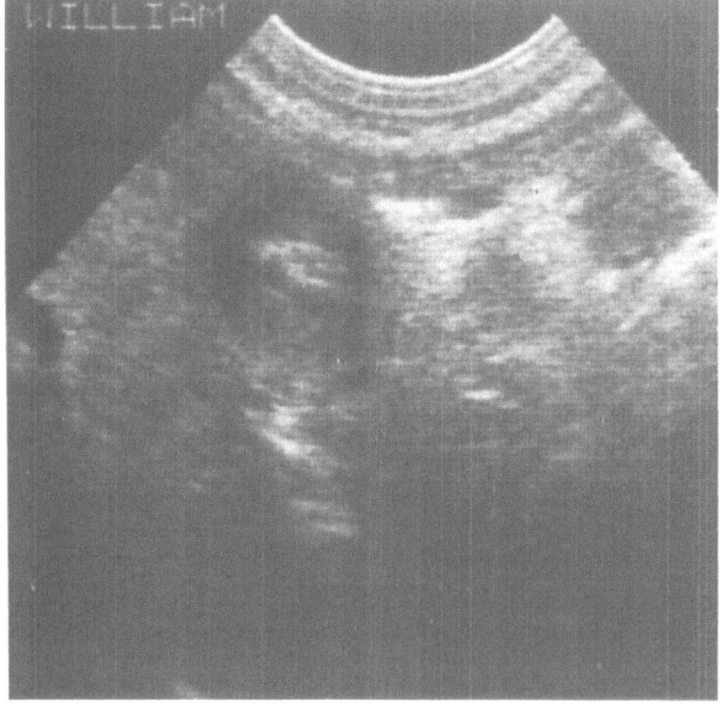

C15.3

Case 16. **This neonate presented at birth with failed passage of a nasogastric tube and was diagnosed as having oesophageal atresia.**

Questions:

1. Describe two significant abnormalities on the supine abdominal radiograph (C16.1).

2. On the chest radiograph (C16.2) a Replogle tube is present in the upper oesophageal pouch.
   a) Describe the lung fields.
   b) Is there a skeletal abnormality?

3. This neonate also has an abnormal left thumb. What other abnormality would you look for?

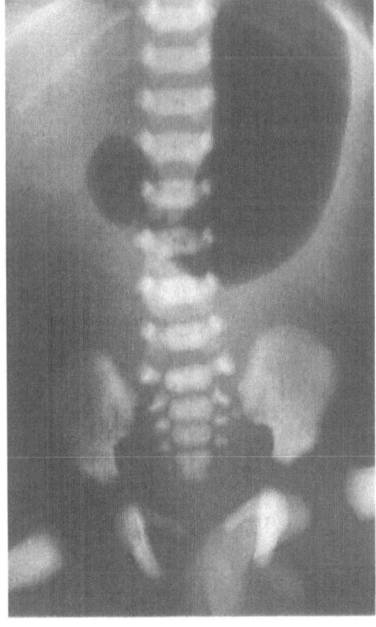

C16.1

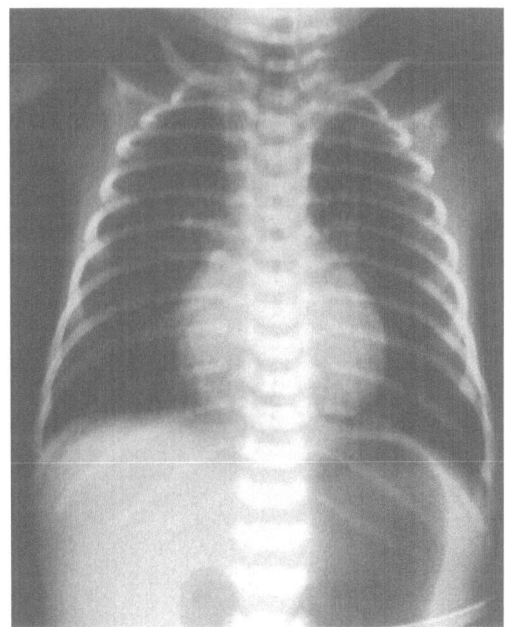

C16.2

Case 16. Answers:

1. a) There is a gas-filled, dilated stomach and first part of duodenum with no gas distally—indicating duodenal atresia.
   b) Six lumbar vertebrae are present.
2. a) The lung fields are plethoric, indicating a left to right shunt.
   b) Thirteen pairs of ribs are present.
3. Renal abnormality (anorectal atresia would be clinically apparent).

Case 16. Comments:

Increased segmentation in the spine is a vertebral abnormality (part of the VATER association) recognised as occurring with oesophageal atresia and anorectal atresia. Decreased segmentation in the thoracic region with only 11 pairs of ribs is a feature of Down's syndrome.

Case 17. This 10-day-old neonate presented with bile stained vomiting.

Questions:

1. Describe the findings on the supine abdominal radiograph (C17.1).
2. What does the barium meal demonstrate (C17.2)?
3. Name three differential diagnoses.

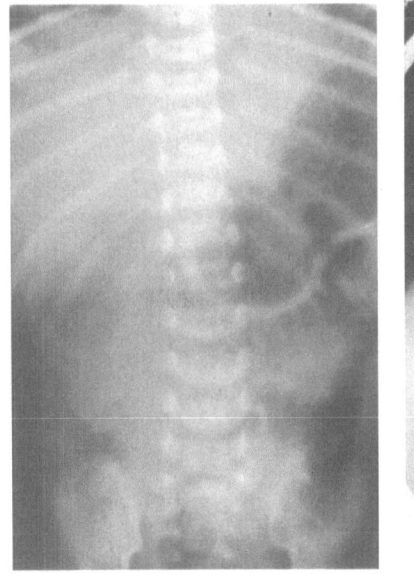

C17.1

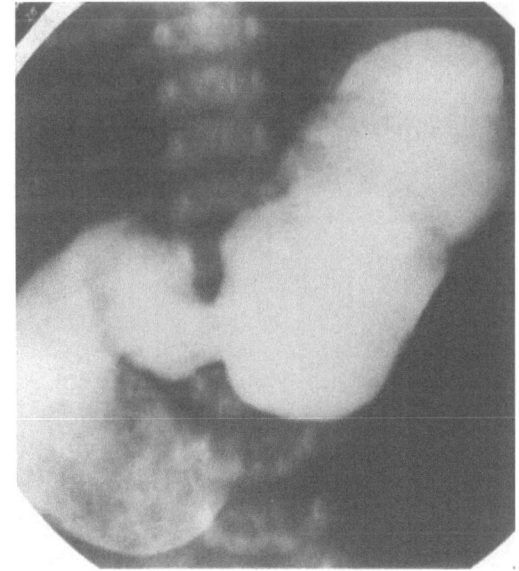

C17.2

Case 17. Answers:

1. Gaseous distension of the stomach and first and second parts of duodenum with some gas present distally.

2. Obstruction in the second part of the duodenum with marked duodenal dilatation and residue.

3. a) Duodenal stenosis (intrinsic or extrinsic annular pancreas).
   b) Duodenal web.
   c) Small-bowel malrotation with volvulus.

Case 17. Comments:

This patient had a duodenal web and the barium meal demonstrates the "windsock" appearance with the web being pushed into the more distal duodenum.

Case 18.   This 10-day-old neonate presented with bile stained vomiting.

Questions:

1. Describe the abnormalities on these straight AP barium meal views (C18.1).
2. What is the diagnosis?
3. Name three major congenital malformations with which this abnormality is usually associated.

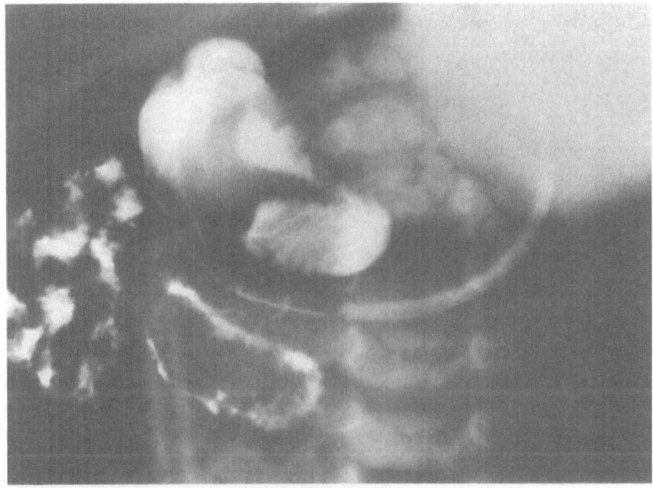

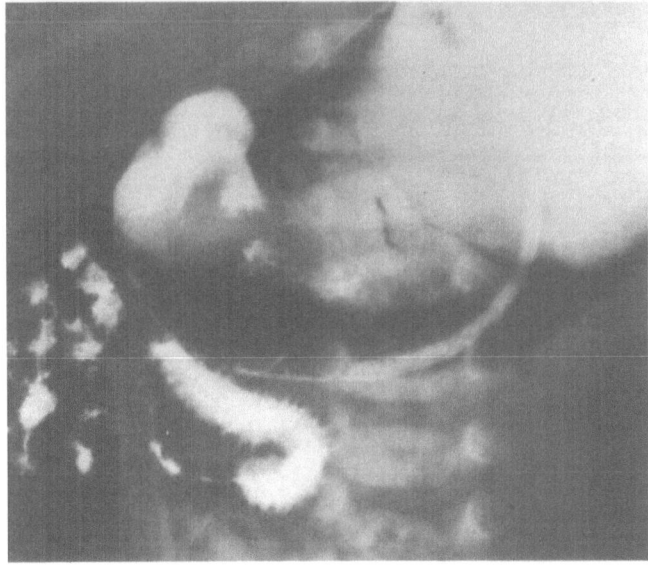

C18.1

Case 18. Answers:

1. The duodeno-jejunal flexure and jejunum lie to the right of the midline.
2. Small-bowel malrotation.
3. a) Congenital Bochdalek-type of diaphragmatic hernia.
   b) Gastroschisis.
   c) Exompholos (omphalocoele).

Case 18. Comments:

On the prone oblique views of the same barium examination (C18.2) there is partial hold-up in the second part of the duodenum. Distal to this, at the site of the volvulus, the duodenum and proximal jejunum appear narrowed—the "twisted-ribbon" sign of a volvulus.

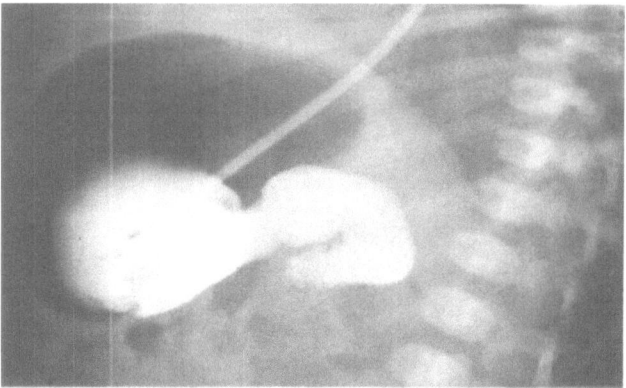

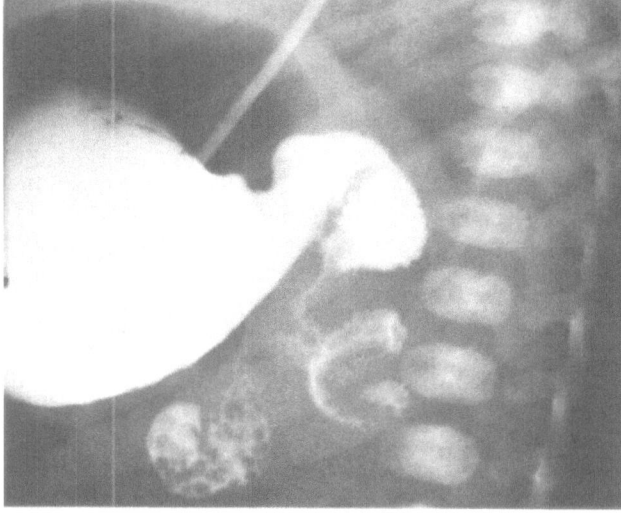

C18.2

Case 19. This 9-month-old infant presented in the Casualty Department after a 12-h history of screaming episodes and intermittent abdominal pain.

Questions:

1. Describe an abnormality on the supine abdominal radiograph (C19.1).
2. What two further examinations would be appropriate?
3. Describe your technique for performing the contrast examination.
4. When do you consider the examination complete?

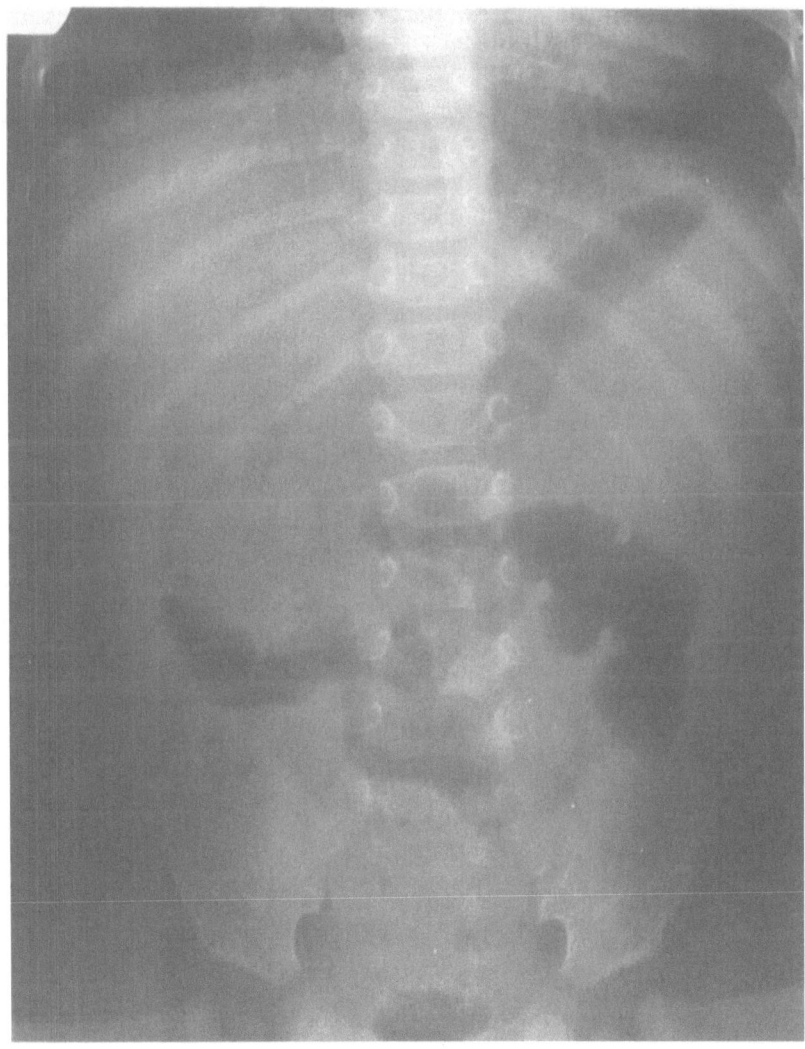

C19.1

Case 19. Answers:

1. A right hypochondral soft tissue mass indents bowel gas in the hepatic flexure.
2. a) Rectal examination to detect the presence of blood.
   b) Barium enema to attempt reduction of intussusception. Examination possible because (i) short history—less than 24 h (ii) no signs of obstruction or peritonism on the radiograph. (No small-bowel dilatation and normal peritoneal fat lines.)
3. Adequate sedation/anaesthesia is needed. (Bowel relaxants are not generally helpful.) Barium introduced under a constant (1 m) head of pressure to prevent perforation, until the head of the intussusception is reached. Pressure maintained until there is reduction.
4. Reduction complete only with free flow into terminal ileum.

Case 19. Comments:

C19.2 illustrates head of intussusception impacted in the caecum.

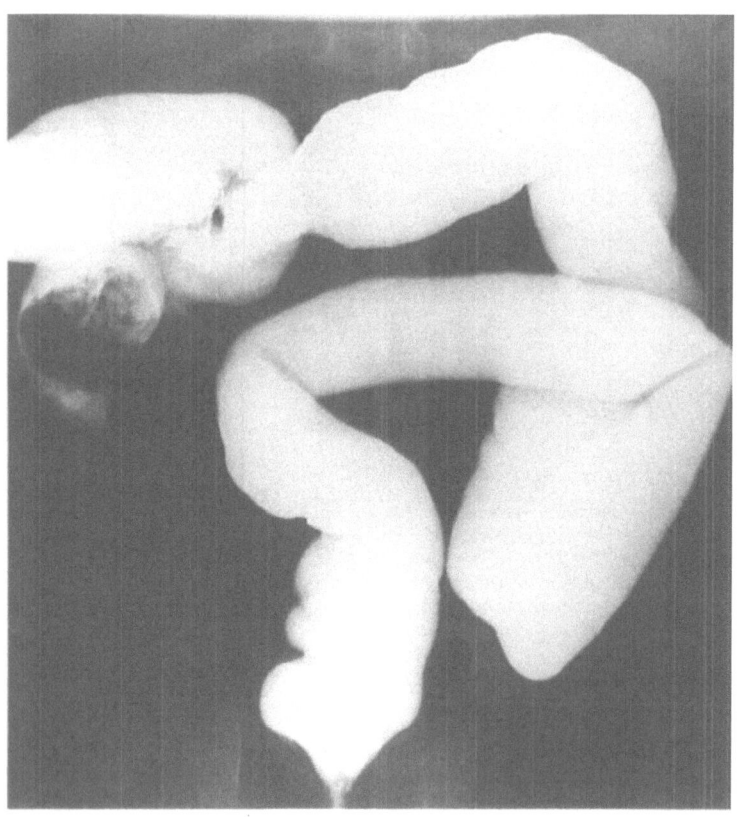

C19.2

Case 20. This 11-year-old girl has had recurrent abdominal pain and she is failing to thrive.

Questions:

1. Describe the abnormalities on the 30-min (C20.1) and 1-h (C20.2) follow-through films of this upper gastro-intestinal series.

2. What is the diagnosis?

3. List the radiological features of a malabsorption pattern.

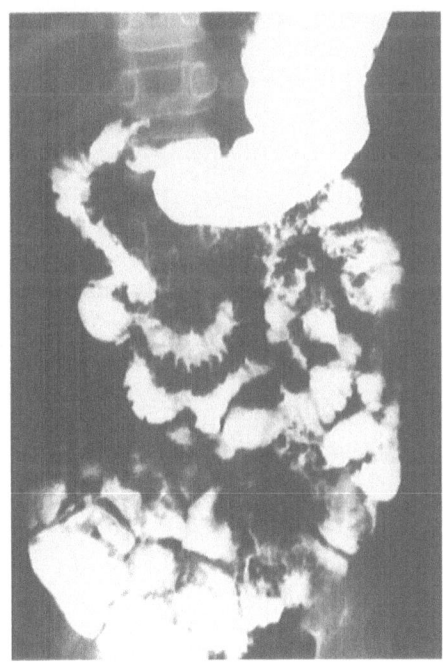 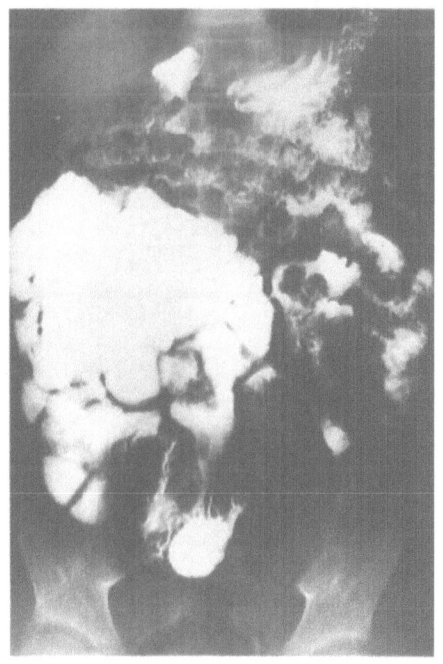

C20.1   C20.2

Case 20. *Answers:*

1. Some ileal and possible asymmetrical pseudodiverticulum formation, thick-ened folds with a "cobblestone" and spiky "rose-thorn" appearance.
2. Crohn's disease.
3. Flocculation and segmentation of the barium column in the ileum, with loss of definition of mucosal folds.

Case 20. *Comments:*

Patients with Crohn's disease usually demonstrate significant retardation of skeletal maturation as assessed by comparing the left hand and wrist with the series compiled by Greulich and Pyle. (These standards are the most widely used method of assessing skeletal maturation, but it should be remembered that the series was compiled from an American population of high social grading and allowances should be made for racial and socio-economic differences.)

Case 21. **This 13-year-old girl presented with anaemia and recurrent abdominal pain.**

Questions:

1. Describe the abnormalities on (a) the supine abdominal radiograph (C21.1) and (b) the ultrasound examination (C21.2).

2. What is the diagnosis?

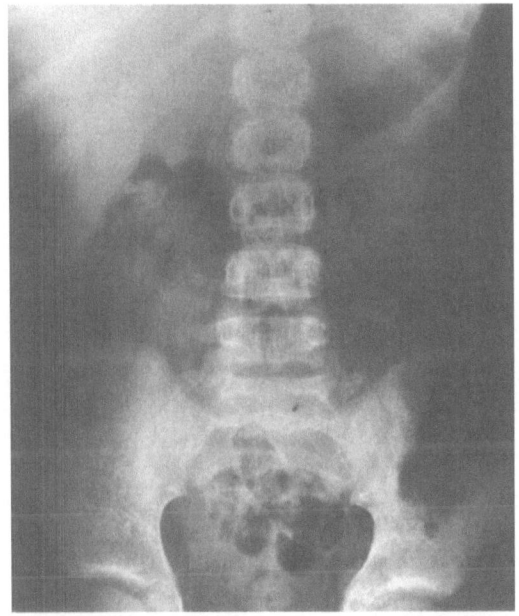

C21.1

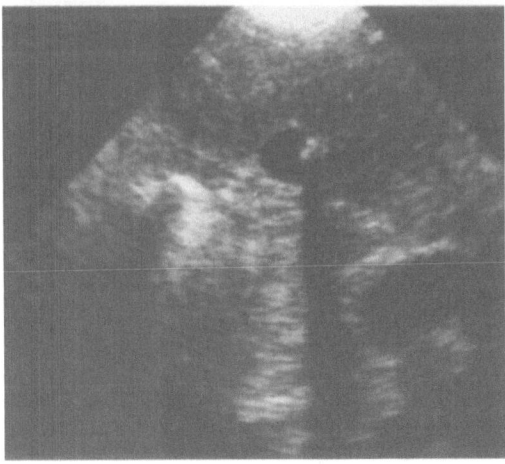

C21.2

Case 21. Answers:

1. a) Osteoporosis with abnormally coarse trabecular pattern throughout and with some bone expansion. The liver is enlarged and there is faecal loading. Several opacities of calcific density are projected over the hepatic flexure.
   b) Acoustic shadows are cast by several gall-stones.

2. Thalassaemia major with bilirubin gall-stones.

Case 22.   This 8-year-old girl presented with an abdominal mass.

Questions:

1. Describe an abnormality of the right kidney on this full length 20-min IVU film (C22.1).
2. What abnormalities would you expect to see on the control film?
3. What is the likely diagnosis?
4. What is the differential diagnosis?
5. What two laboratory tests would help to elucidate the problem?

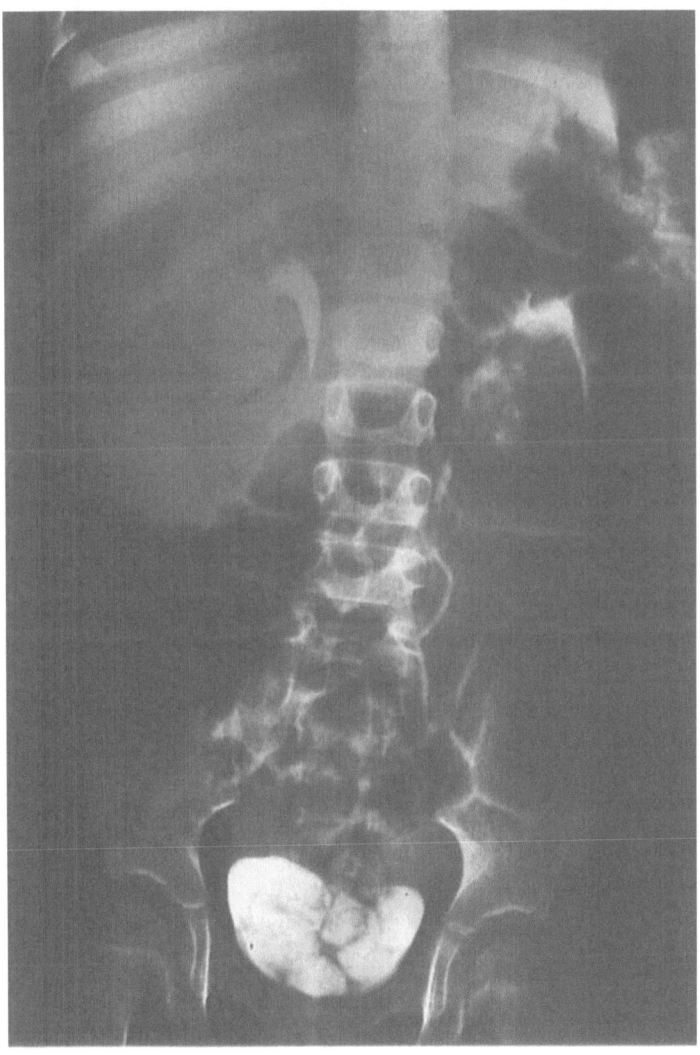

C22.1

Case 22. Answers:

1. Displaced upwards.

2. Right hypochondral soft tissue mass with speckled malignant tumour calcification.

3. Hepatoblastoma because the calcification/mass is probably in the liver.

4. Neuroblastoma (most are above the kidney and would displace it downwards). Wilms' tumour (nephroblastoma) would be unlikely because of absence of distortion of the pelvi-calyceal system and the presence of calcification.

5. Alpha-fetoproteins raised in hepatoblastoma. VMA raised in neuroblastoma.

Case 23.   This 1-year-old girl presented with a right-sided abdominal mass.

Questions:

1. Describe the appearances of the right kidney on this 10-min IVU film (C23.1).
2. What soft tissue abnormality would you see on the control film of the IVU series?
3. What is the differential diagnosis?
4. What further studies would be indicated and why?

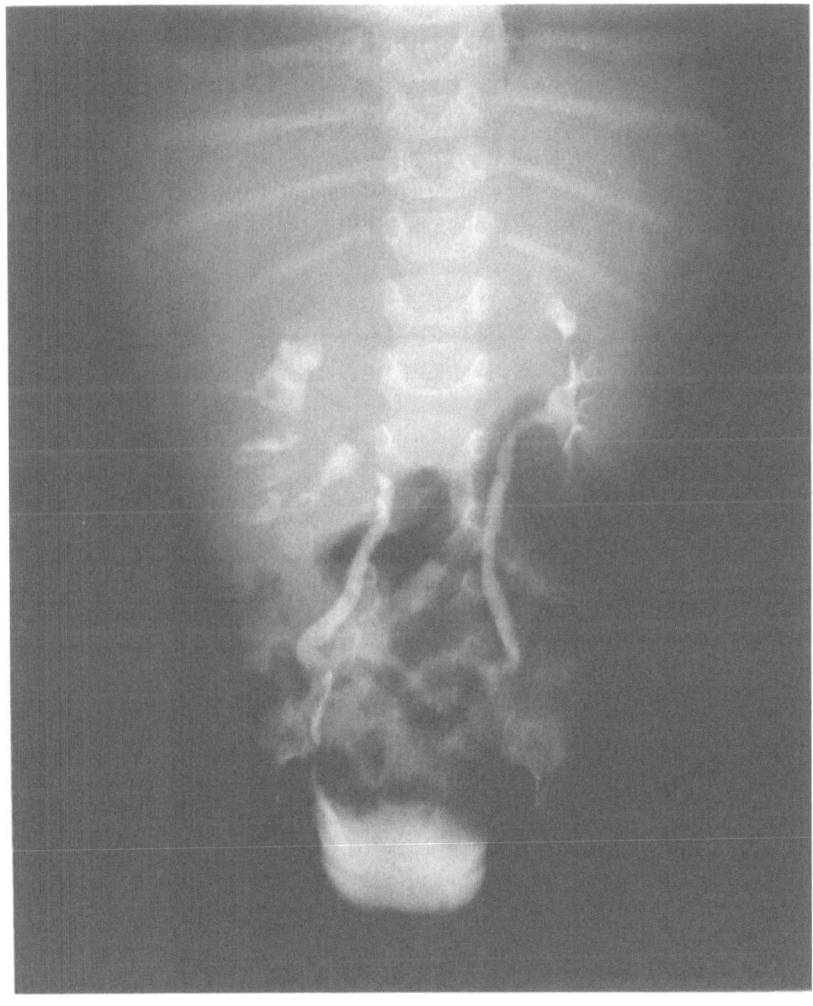

C23.1

Case 23. Answers:

1. The right renal outline is larger than the left. It is low and the calyces are distorted. The changes result from extrinsic compression.

2. An enlarged liver.

3. Hepatoblastoma (final diagnosis), hepatocellular carcinoma, hepatoma, A-V malformation, abscess.

4. a) Ultrasound—confirm hepatic mass; assess involvement.
   b) Computed tomography—as above.
   c) Selective hepatic angiography—determines vascular anatomy and supply pre-operatively.
   d) Alpha-fetoproteins (elevated in hepatoblastoma).

Case 23. Comments:

Transverse ultrasound scan (C23.2) shows mixed increased and decreased echo pattern of lobulated hepatic masses. Computed tomography (C23.3) shows a low density mass in right lobe of liver. A hepatic angiogram (digital subtraction angiography) in the arterial phase (C23.4) shows a normal left hepatic artery, but stretched and abnormal branches on the right.

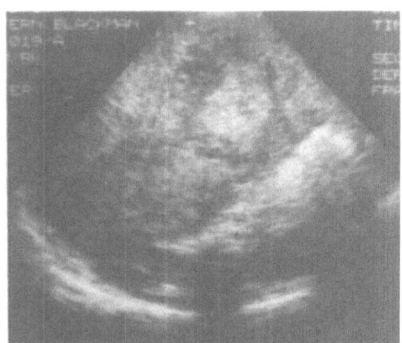

C23.2

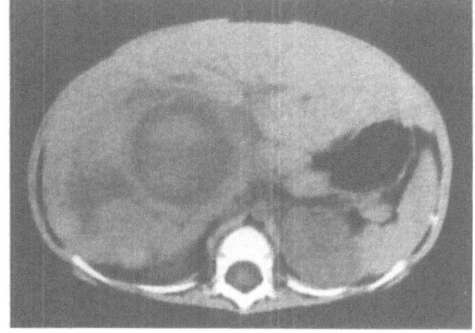

C23.3

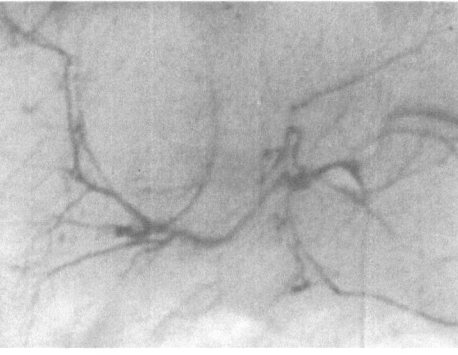

C23.4

Case 24. This 2-year-old boy presented with an abdominal mass.

Questions:

1. What abnormalities are demonstrated on this 30-min IVU film (C24.1)?
2. What is the likely diagnosis?

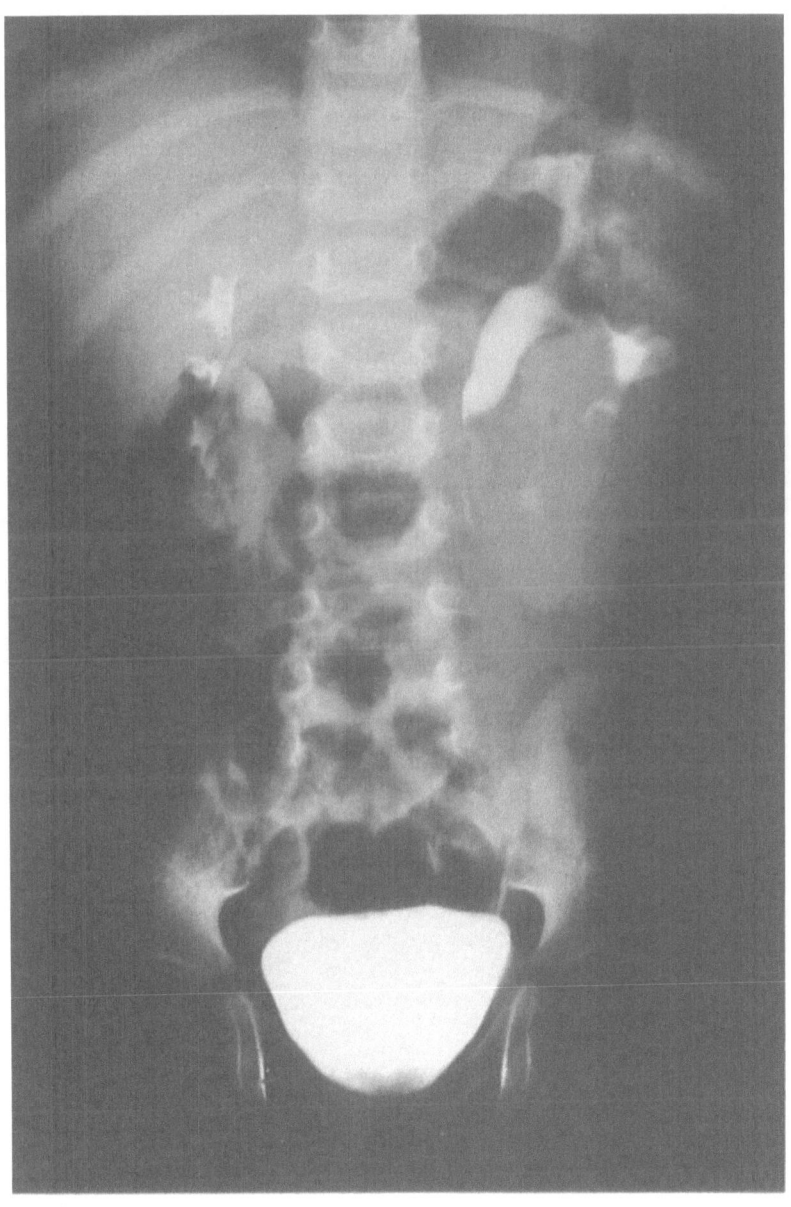

C24.1

Case 24. *Answers:*

1. There is a large left kidney with distortion of the pelvi-calyceal system, indicating an intrarenal mass lesion.

2. Wilms' tumour (nephroblastoma).

Case 24. *Comments:*

In Wilms' tumour calcification is uncommon (less than 10%) but if present it may be punctate or curvilinear. Wilms' tumour rarely crosses the midline. Spread across the midline is more common in neuroblastoma. Renal ultrasound demonstrates a mixed echo pattern. C24.2 (longitudinal left renal ultrasound scan) illustrates a left upper pole Wilms' tumour with evidence of the characteristic transonic "lakes" best seen between the accoustic rib shadows.

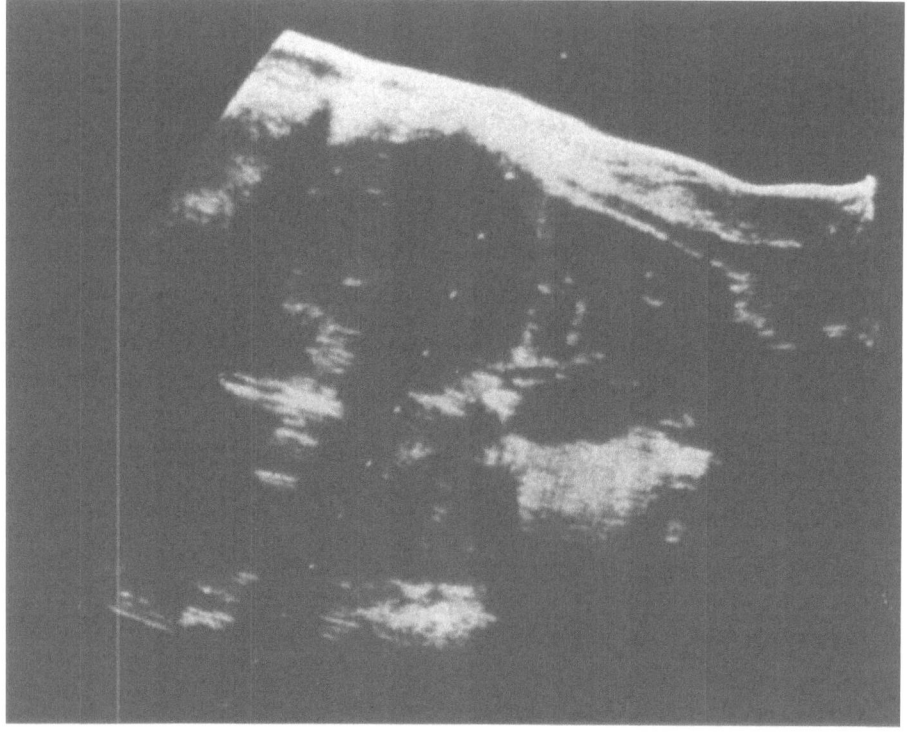

C24.2

Case 25. **This 5-year-old girl presented with a urinary tract infection and some haematuria.**

Questions:

1. Describe the renal abnormalities on the 15-min full length IVU film (C25.1).

2. What is the differential diagnosis?

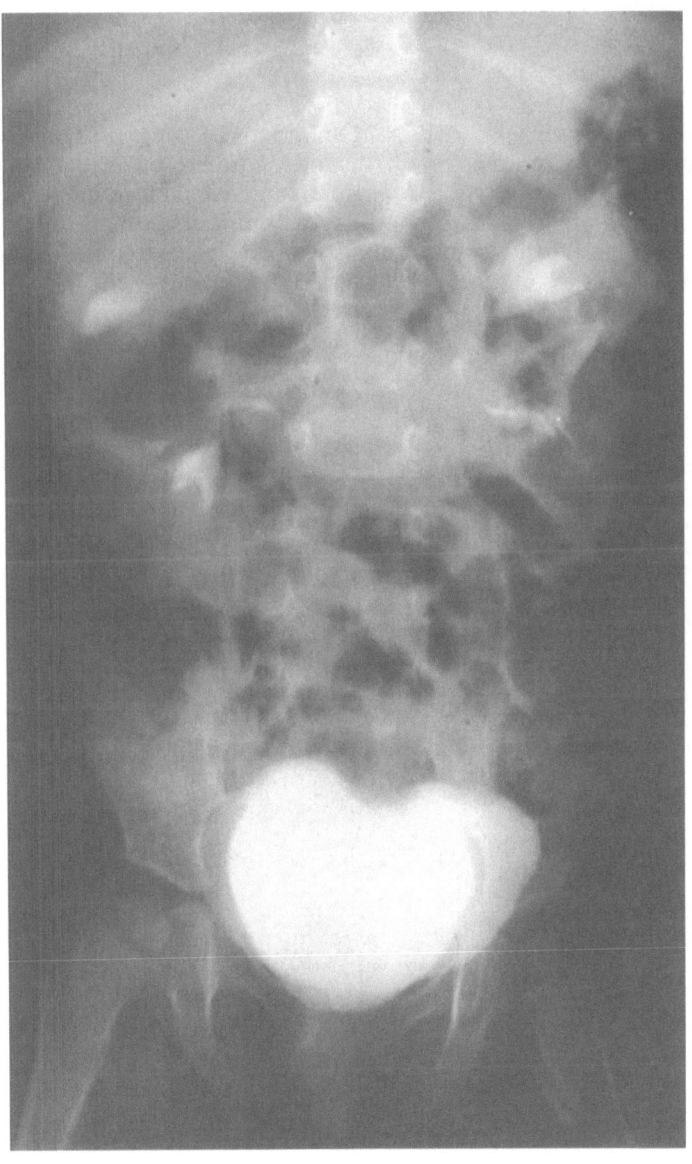

C25.1

Case 25.   Answers:

1. Both kidneys are enlarged. The calyces are distorted and splayed and there is stretching and compression of the infundibula. These appearances are caused by bilateral intrarenal space-occupying lesions. In addition there is a rounded negative nephrogram in the right upper pole (projected over the liver) indicating a cyst here.

2. Adult-type of polycystic disease.
   Tuberose sclerosis (final diagnosis).
   Rare forms of bilateral cystic dysplastic kidneys.

Case 25.   Comments:

Adult polycystic disease (autosomal dominant inheritance) may present in childhood and has been shown in utero on ultrasound. In tuberose sclerosis the kidneys contain a combination of cysts and angiomyolipoma. The lipomatous element may be demonstrated on plain tomography as transradiant areas of less than soft tissue density due to the low atomic number of fat. Bony abnormalities may also be evident (C25.2) as multiple focal areas of sclerosis.

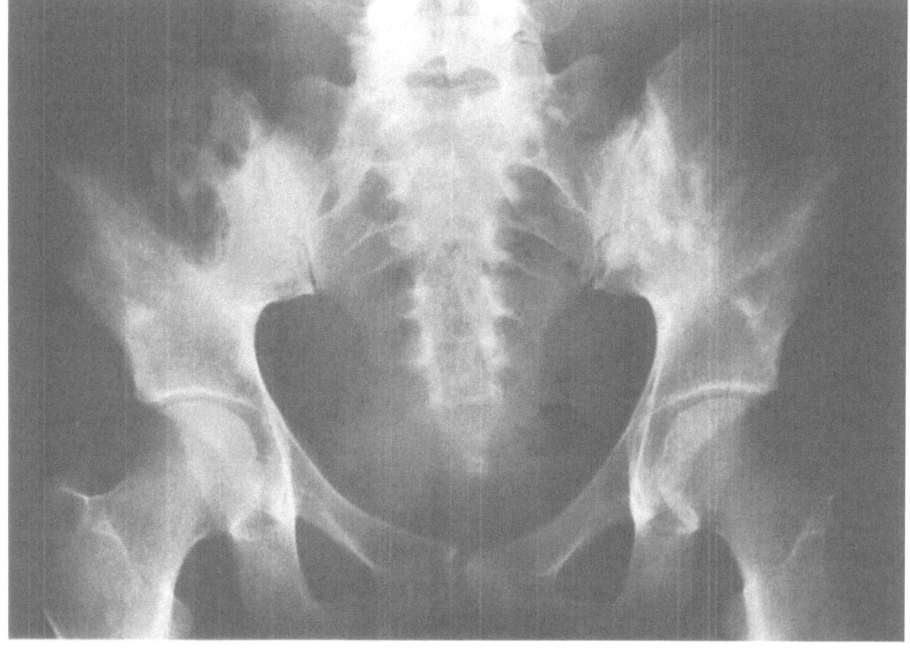

C25.2

Case 26. **This neonate presented with abdominal distension and palpable kidneys.**

Questions:

1. Describe the changes on this 4-h IVU film (C26.1).
2. What is the contrast medium of choice?
3. What is the diagnosis and prognosis?

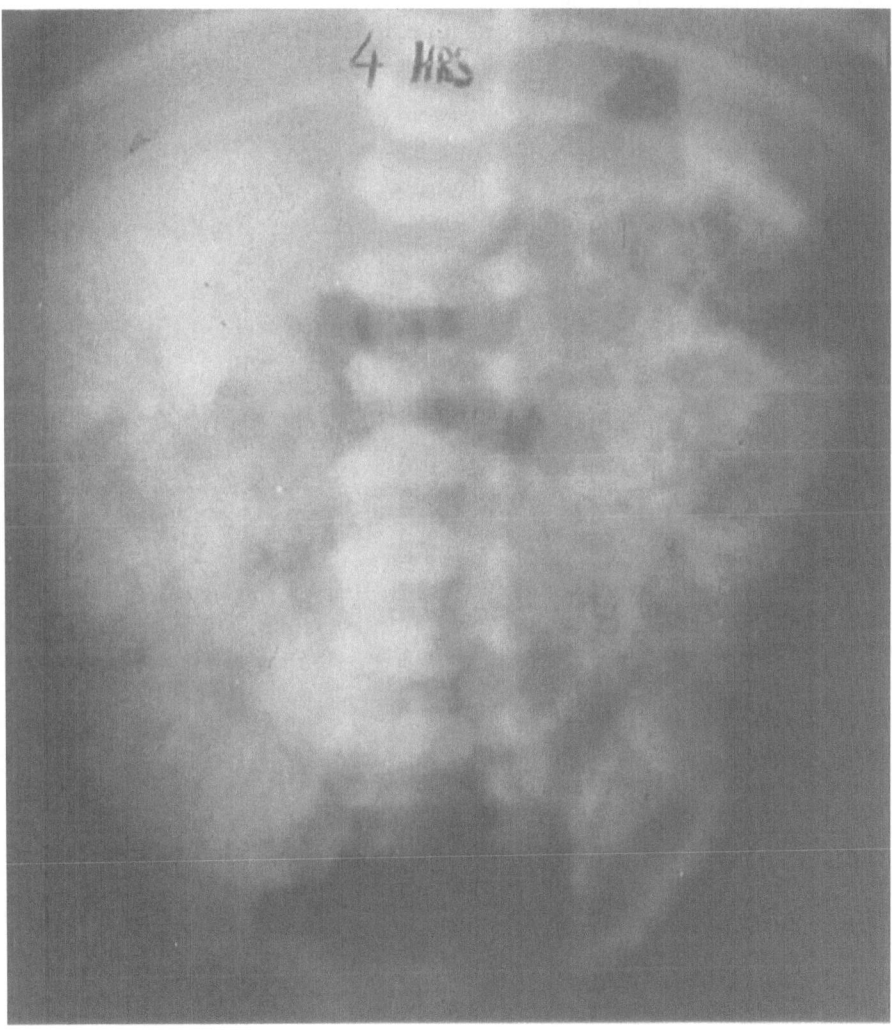

C26.1

Case 26. *Answers:*

1. Both kidneys are enlarged with radiating streaks of opacification throughout the cortex. The pelvi-calyceal systems have not been filled.

2. Non-ionic contrast.

3. Infantile polycystic disease (autosomal recessive inheritance). When presenting in the neonatal period the prognosis is very poor.

Case 26. *Comments:*

The DTPA renogram (C26.2) illustrates excretion by both kidneys which appear to occupy the entire abdomen.

C26.3 illustrates the typical bright echo pattern seen on ultrasound. Macroscopic cysts are not present.

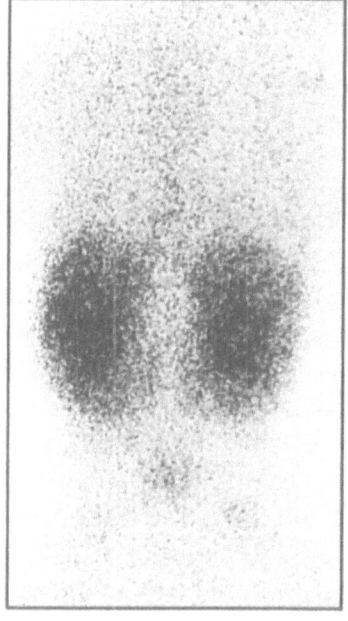

C26.2

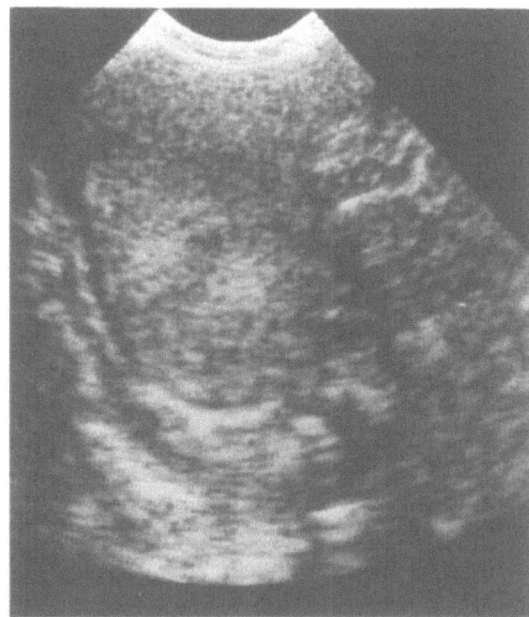

C26.3

Case 27. This female infant presented with abdominal distension and two palpably enlarged kidneys; she had passed very little urine since birth.

Questions:

1. Describe the appearances of the transverse (C27.1) and longitudinal (C27.2) ultrasound scans of the left renal area.

2. What is the diagnosis?

3. Why might the right kidney be enlarged?

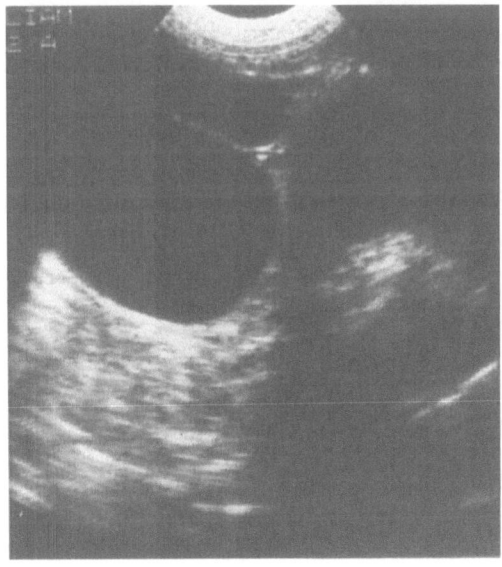

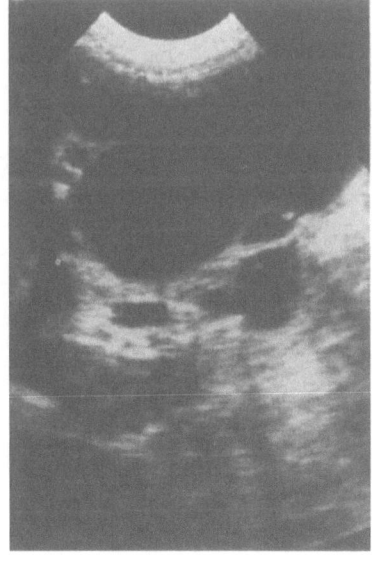

C27.1   C27.2

Case 27. Answers:

1. There are multiple rounded echolucent areas of differing sizes which do not connect with each other and there is virtually no evidence of normal renal parenchyma.

2. Multicystic kidney.

3. Thirty-three per cent of patients with multicystic kidneys have other congenital renal anomalies.

C27.3, taken 3 h following an intravenous contrast injection, illustrates the right-sided pelvi-ureteric junction obstruction, with no excretion on the side of the multicystic kidney.

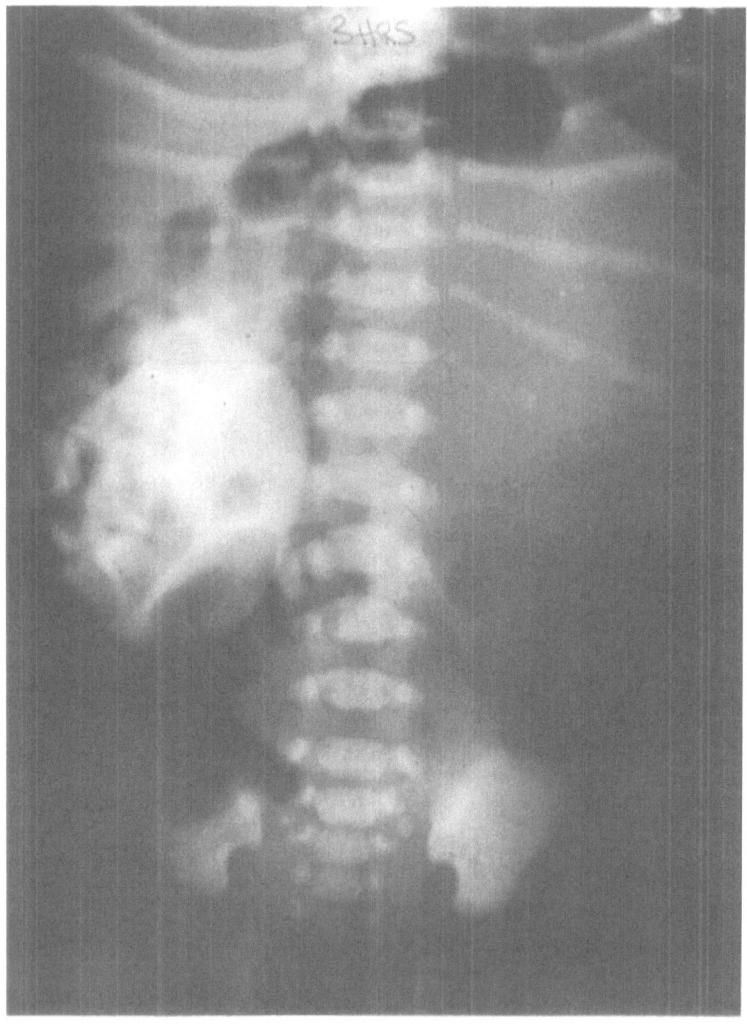

C27.3

Case 28. A 4-year-old boy presented with recurrent left loin pain.

Questions:

1. Describe the left kidney as seen on this 1-h IVU film (C28.1).
2. Why is the axis of the left kidney altered?
3. What is the diagnosis?
4. What additional information would a DTPA renogram give?

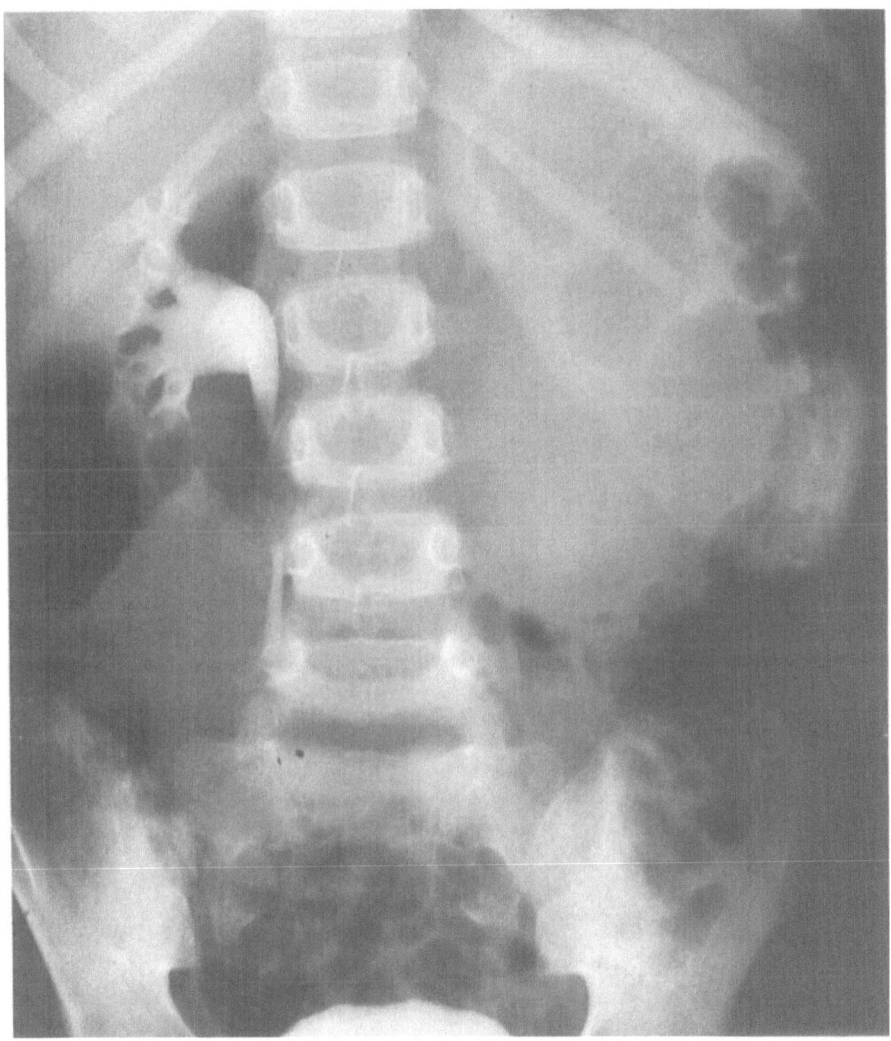

C28.1

Case 28. *Answers:*

1. Hydronephrosis with a dense rim nephrogram and a crescent appearance around "negative" dilated calyces.

2. The hugely dilated renal pelvis (soft tissue opacity to the left of L3–L4) displaces the lower pole laterally.

3. Obstruction at pelvi-ureteric junction level.

4. Differential function of the two kidneys. It would also help to confirm the presence and level of obstruction. C28.2 illustrates an isotope renogram 10 min after intravenous DTPA, C28.3 10 min following intravenous frusemide. There has been wash-out on the normal right side but the left pelvis has further enlarged and shows no reduction in activity, confirming obstruction. C28.4 illustrates the activity curves.

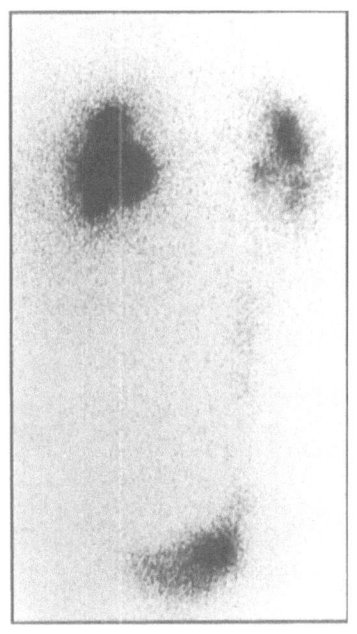 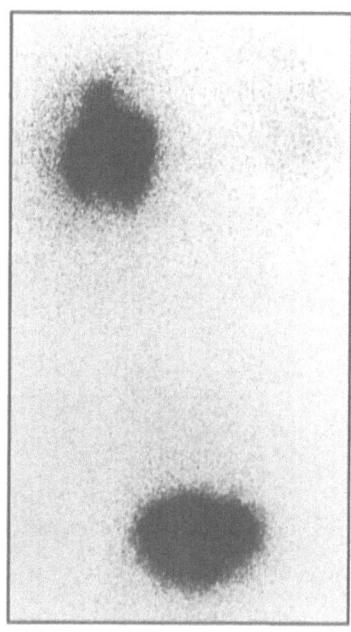

C28.2   C28.3

C28.4

Case 29. This 4-month-old girl presented with a urinary tract infection.

Questions:

1. Describe the appearances of the bladder on the late IVU film (C29.1).
2. Describe the appearances on the midline longitudinal ultrasound scan of the bladder (C29.2).
3. What is the diagnosis?
4. What would you expect to see in the upper renal tracts?

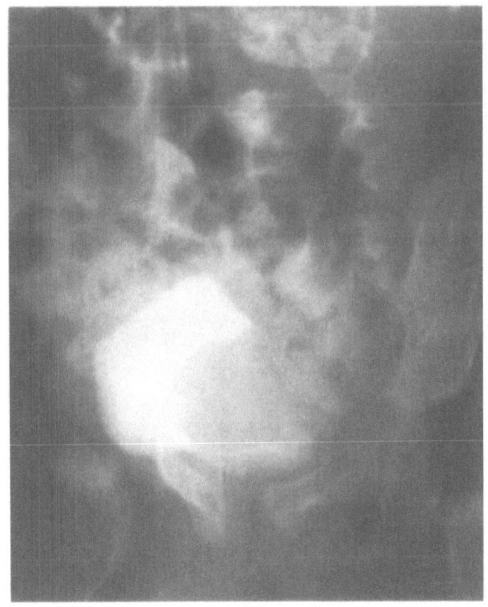

C29.1

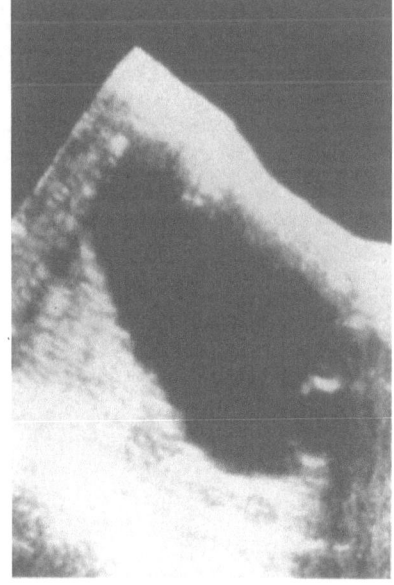

C29.2

Case 29. Answers:

1. Large left-sided intrinsic filling defect in the bladder.
2. Transonic rounded defect in the bladder base.
3. Ureterocoele.
4. Duplex system on the left with obstructed upper moiety.

Case 29. Comments:

IVU film (C29.3) shows non-functioning upper moiety of a left duplex system (lower moiety calyces too few and too far from spine to be a normal kidney). A right duplex system is also present.

C29.4 shows a longitudinal ultrasound scan of the left kidney. Transonic non-functioning upper moiety of duplex kidney.

C29.5 shows a left longitudinal ultrasound scan of bladder. Dilated, obstructed left ureter behind bladder.

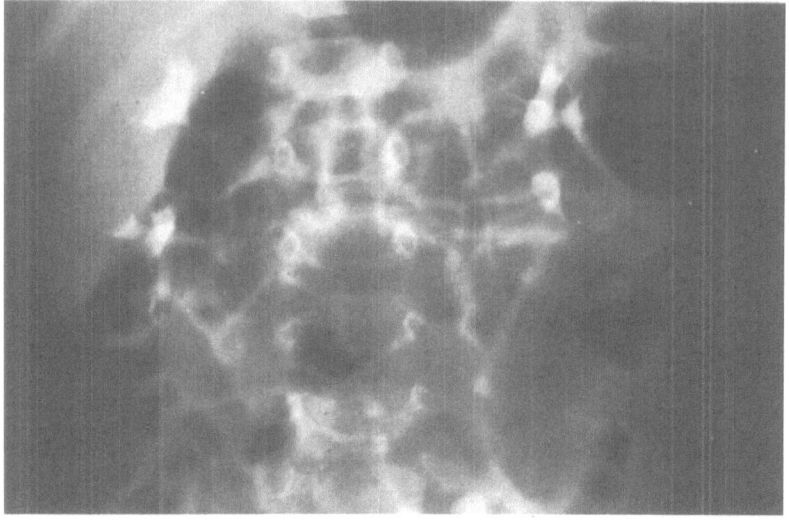

C29.3

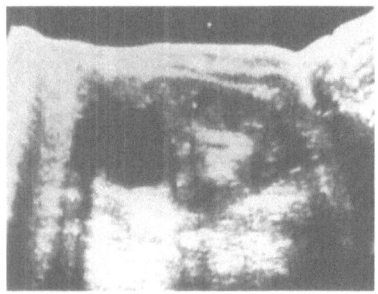

C29.4

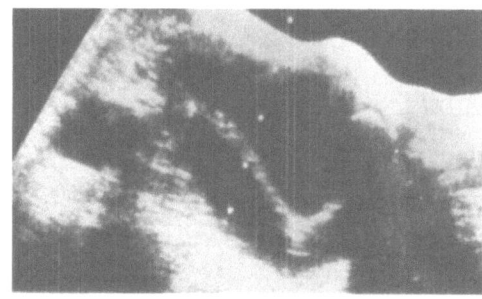

C29.5

Case 30. This 18-month-old girl presented with recurrent urinary tract infections and difficulty with micturition.

Questions:

1. Describe the abnormality on these three views of a micturating cystourethrography series (C30.1).
2. What is the likely diagnosis?
3. What would you expect to see in the kidneys on (a) an IVU and (b) a DTPA renogram?

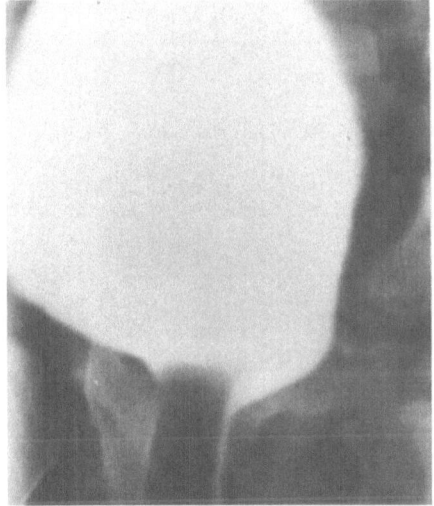

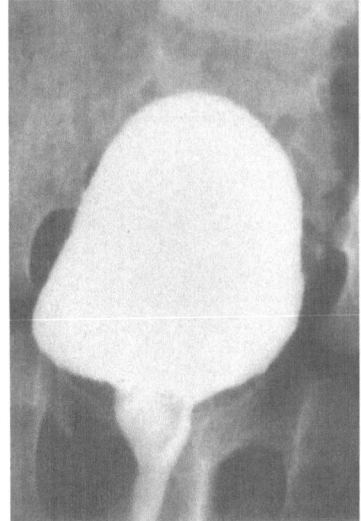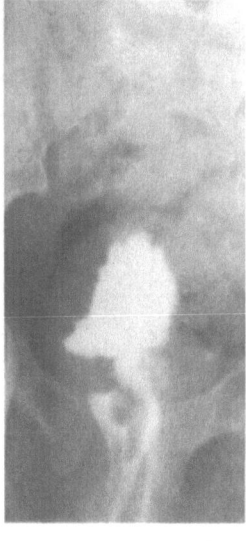

C30.1

Case 30. *Answers:*

1. There is a constant filling defect in the bladder base and urethra.
2. Prolapsing ectopic ureterocoele (possible blood clot or rhabdomyosarcoma).
3. a) Obstructed upper moeity of a duplex system (C30.2).
   b) Non-functioning or poorly functioning obstructed upper pole of a kidney (C30.3).

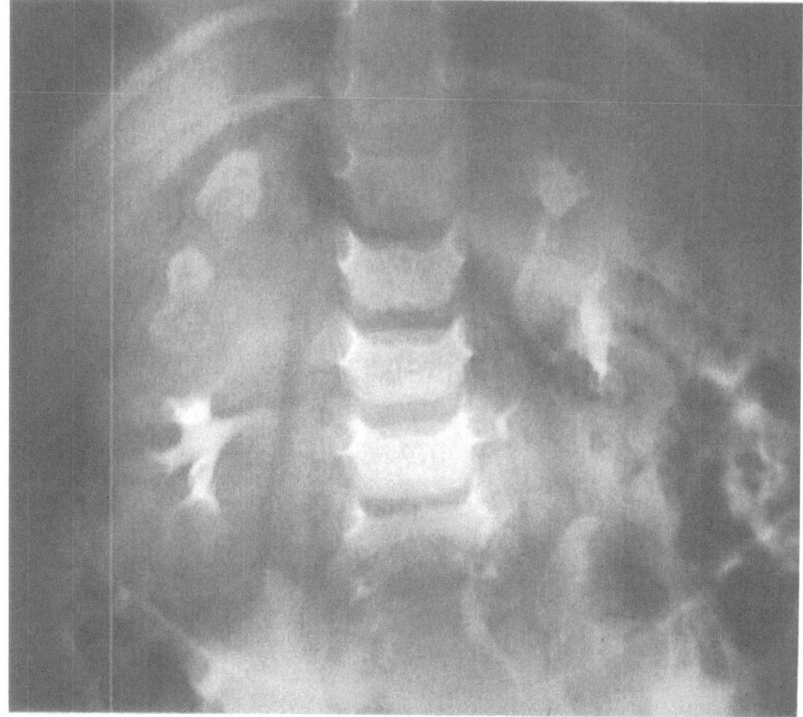

C30.2

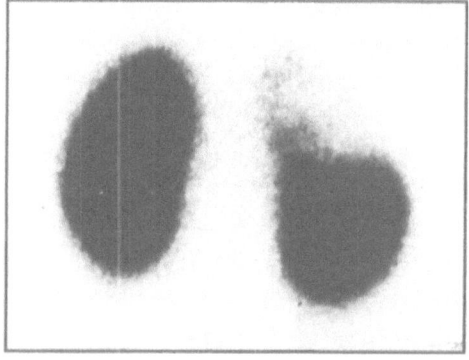

C30.3

Case 31. This 3-year-old boy presented with recurrent urinary tract infections.

Questions:

1. On this 1-h IVU film (C31.1) give one word to describe:
   a) The kidneys.
   b) The ureters.
2. What is the differential diagnosis?
3. What investigation would you request now?

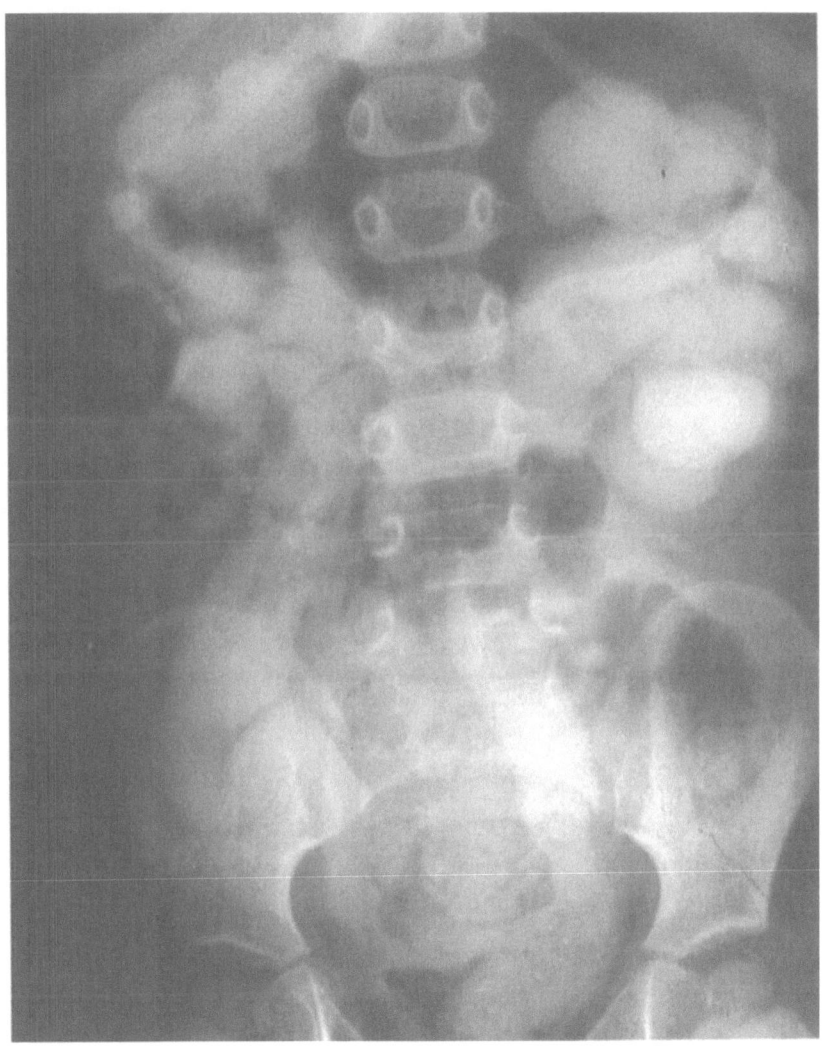

C31.1

Case 31. Answers:

1. a) Hydronephroses.
   b) Hydroureters.

2. a) Bladder outflow obstruction (posterior urethral valves or neurogenic bladder).
   b) Congenital megaureters with bilateral obstruction at uretero-vesical junctions.

3. Micturating cystourethrogram to demonstrate posterior urethral valves or a neurogenic bladder.

Case 32. **This neonate presented with failure to pass urine and palpable kidneys.**

Questions:

1. Describe the changes on the two urethral views of the micturating cystogram (C32.1).
2. What is the diagnosis?
3. What renal abnormalities might you find in this condition?

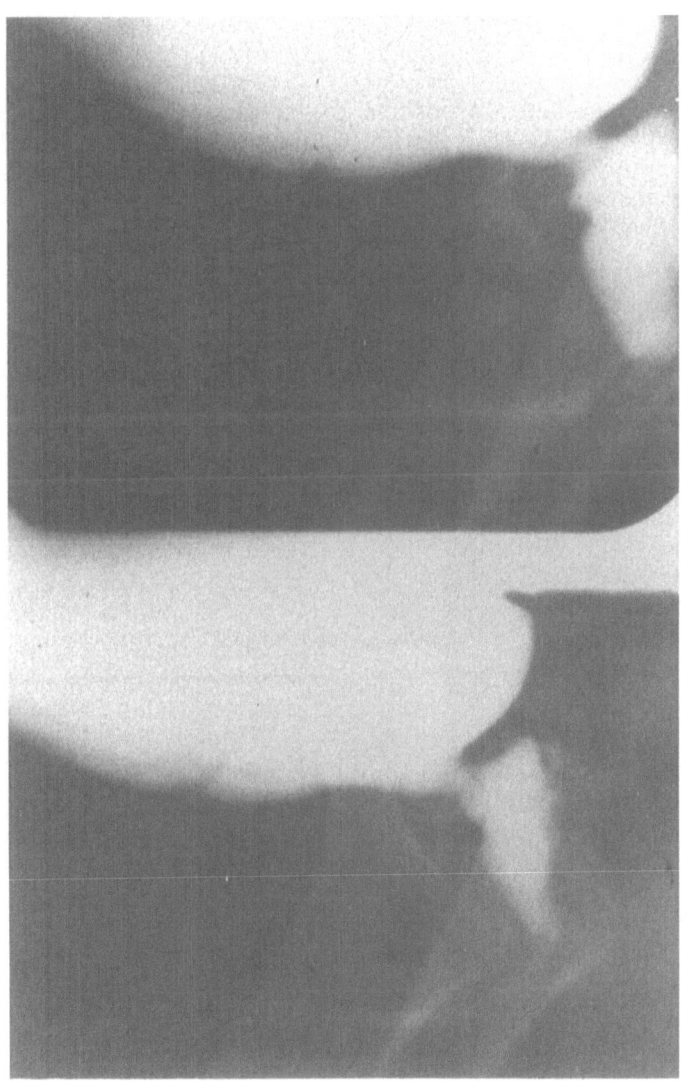

C32.1

Case 32. *Answers:*

1. The posterior urethra is dilated with a little filling of prostatic ducts. There is a poor stream through the anterior urethra.

2. Posterior urethral valves.

3. a) Hydronephroses due to reflux or secondary uretero-vesical junction obstruction due to bladder wall thickening.
   b) Intrarenal reflux due to back pressure.
   c) Parenchymal cystic changes due to primary renal dysplasia.
   d) Ruptured fornix of an upper pole calyx causing urinary ascites or a urinoma.

Case 32. *Comments:*

Voiding views without a catheter in position are necessary to demonstrate obstruction at the valve site. C32.2 is an AP view demonstrating valve and dilated posterior urethra; thick-walled bladder; bilateral reflux; right hydronephrosis with intraparenchymal cysts. C32.3 shows reflux and hydronephrosis with intrarenal reflux.

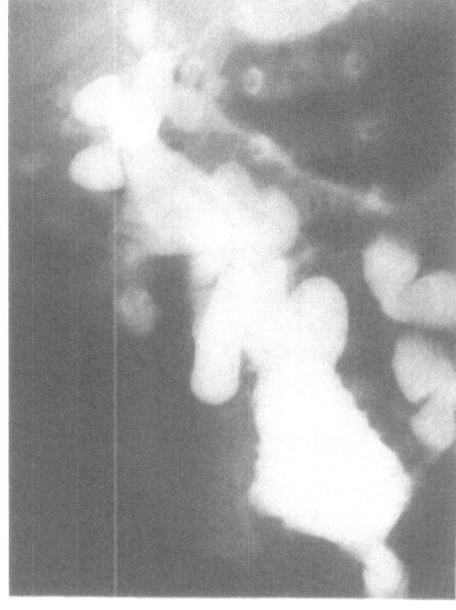

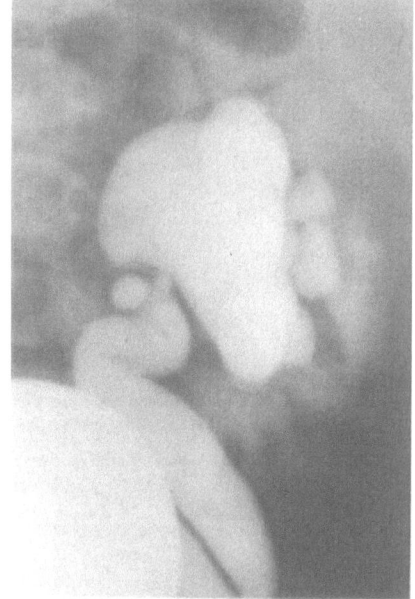

C32.2   C32.3

Case 33. This 3-year-old boy presented with recurrent urinary tract infections.

Questions:

1. What abnormalities are demonstrated on the micturating cystourethrogram (C33.1)?
2. What would you expect to see on ultrasound of the kidneys?

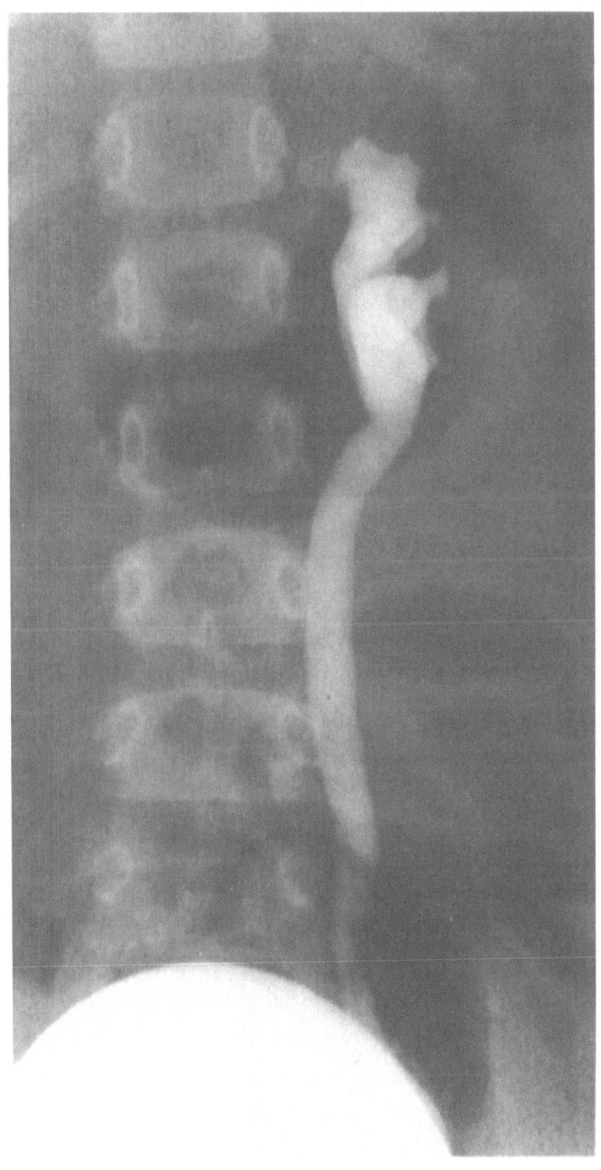

C33.1

Case 33. *Answers:*

1. There is left-sided reflux into a moderately dilated ureter and into the pelvicalyceal system. There is loss of normal calyceal cupping.

2. The right kidney shows compensatory hypertrophy and measures 8.2 cm (C33.2). The left kidney is small as a result of reflux and pyelonephritis and measures 4.3 cm (C33.3).

Case 33. *Comments:*

Cortical scarring may be difficult to demonstrate on ultrasound but is well demonstrated on a DMSA radionuclide scan. Causes of a small kidney without hydronephrosis include pyelonephritis, old renal vein thrombosis and renal artery stenosis.

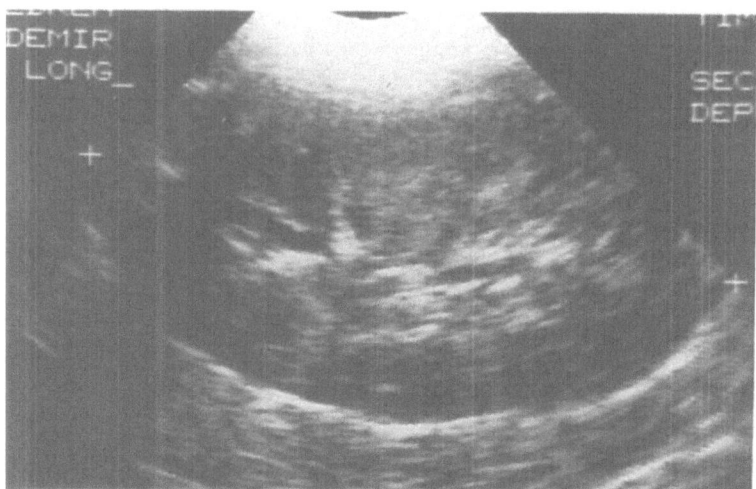

C33.2

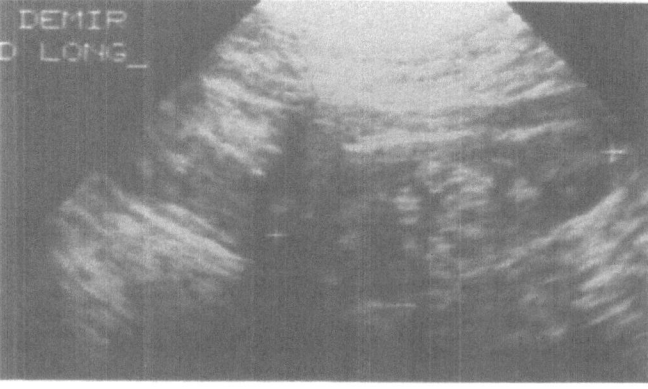

C33.3

Case 34. **This 5-year-old girl presented with urinary tract infections. She was known to have spinal dysraphism.**

Questions:

1. Describe the renal abnormality on this full length 15-min IVU film (C34.1).

2. What complications may be associated with this condition?

3. There is abnormal widening of the interpedicular distances in the lower lumbar spine, reflecting spinal dysraphism. Describe one other skeletal abnormality.

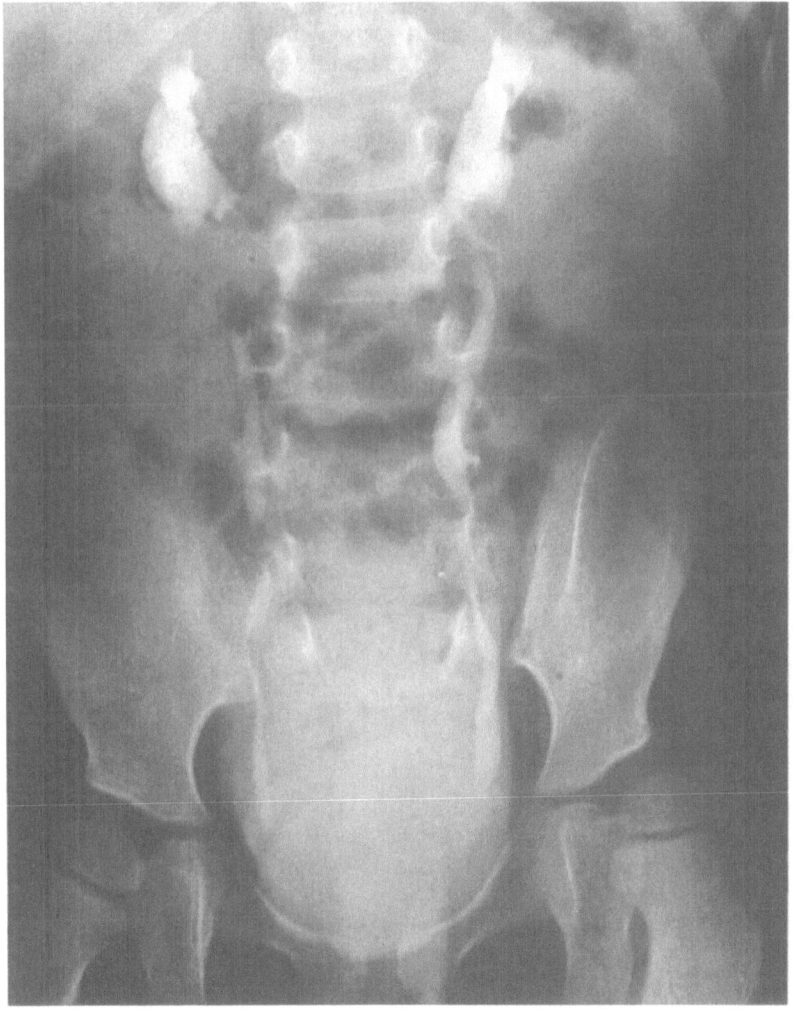

C34.1

Case 34. Answers:

1. The axes of the pelvi-calyceal systems are rotated so that the lower poles lie medially, suggesting a horse-shoe kidney.

2. Infection; obstruction at pelvi-ureteric junction level; calculus formation.

3. Both acetabular roofs are shallow and slope steeply and the capital femoral epiphyses are incompletely covered (subluxation of both hips).

Case 34. Comments:

The IVU performed 4 years later (C34.2) demonstrates dilatated renal pelves with blunted calyces. Both ureters are dilated and the bladder poorly opacified. This suggests partial obstruction—at the pelvi-ureteric junction level and at the vesico-ureteric junction due to thickened neurogenic bladder wall. C34.3 is a DTPA renogram. Functioning renal tissue crosses midline. Obstruction confirmed by long mean transit times and poor response to frusemide.

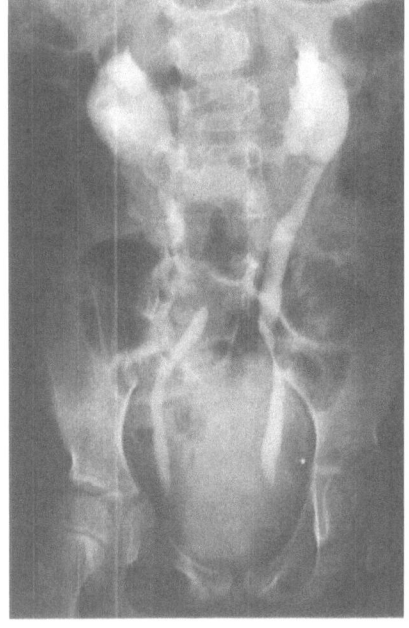

C34.2

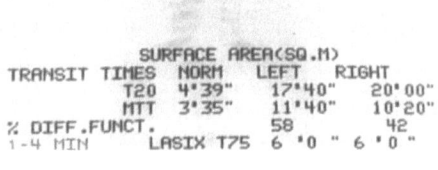

TRANSIT TIMES	SURFACE AREA(SQ.M) NORM	LEFT	RIGHT
T20	4'39"	17'40"	20'00"
MTT	3'35"	11'40"	10'20"
% DIFF.FUNCT.		58	42
1-4 MIN	LASIX T75	6 '0 "	6 '0 "

C34.3

Case 35. This 4-year-old girl had recurrent urinary tract infections. She has had a ventriculo-peritoneal shunt inserted.

Questions:

1. Describe three significant skeletal abnormalities on the control film of an IVU series (C35.1).
2. Describe the appearances on the cystogram (C35.2).
3. What are the bladder changes due to?

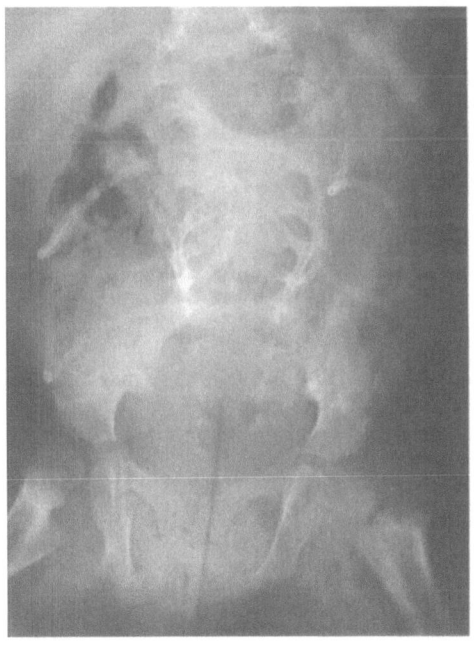

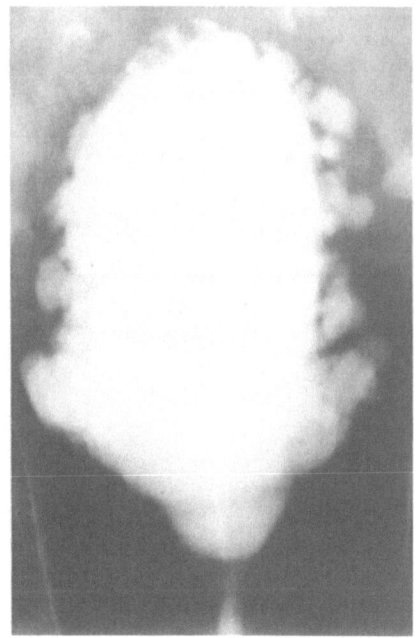

C35.1   C35.2

Case 35. Answers:

1. a) There is spinal dysraphism extending downwards from the lower dorsal spine.
   b) The acetabula are shallow and poorly formed.
   c) There is irregularity and broadening of the left femoral neck with some cortical thickening of the shaft. Changes of an old neuropathic fracture.

2. The bladder is small-volumed and elongated (pine-cone appearance). The wall is thickened and trabeculated with multiple diverticula. The bladder neck is wide.

3. Outflow obstruction due to a neuropathic bladder.

Case 36. This 6-month-old girl presented with progressive abdominal distension and straining on micturition.

Questions:

1. Describe the appearances on the supine abdominal radiograph (C36.1).

2. Describe the abnormalities on the transverse (C36.2) and longitudinal (C36.3) ultrasound scans of the pelvis.

3. What other imaging investigation may be of value?

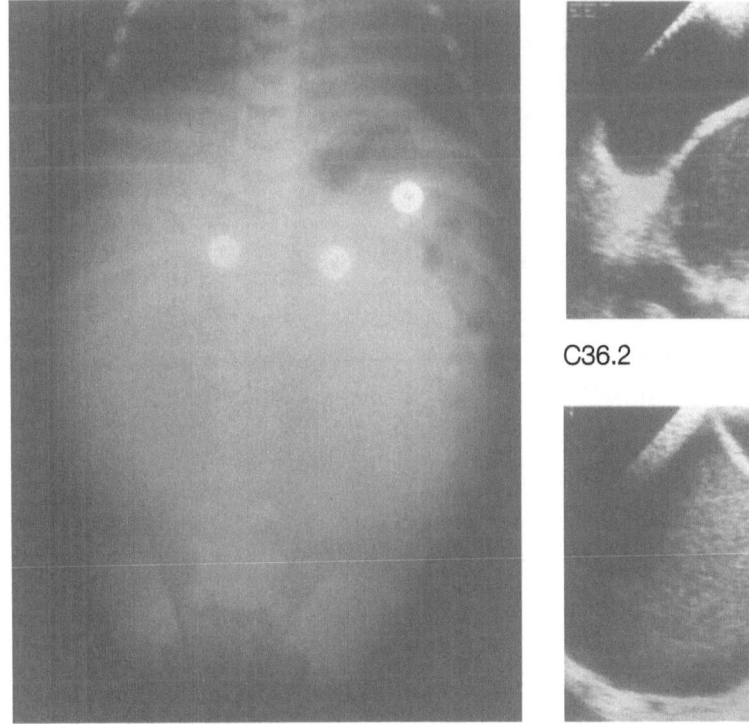

C36.2

C36.1   C36.3

71

Case 36. Answers:

1. The abdomen is distended. Bowel gas shadows are displaced upwards and into the left flank by a soft tissue mass.

2. The bladder (transonic) is compressed and displaced forwards by a large, walled cystic mass which lies within the pelvis and abdomen.

3. Computed tomography.

Case 36. Comments:

The child has a hydrometrocolpos. C36.4 demonstrates the computed tomographic scans—transversely through the pelvis with changes similar to those seen on the ultrasound examination and longitudinally demonstrating the pelvic origin of the large intra abdominal mass. Large ovarian masses usually rise out of the pelvis.

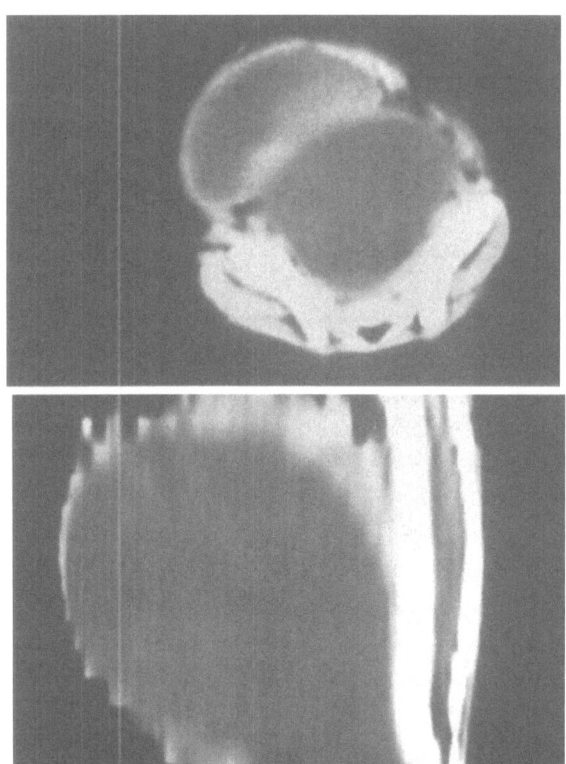

C36.4

Case 37. This is the first chest radiograph (C37.1) taken at 10 h in a full-term baby with respiratory distress since birth.

Questions:

1. Describe two significant abnormalities.
2. What could be the cause of the respiratory distress?

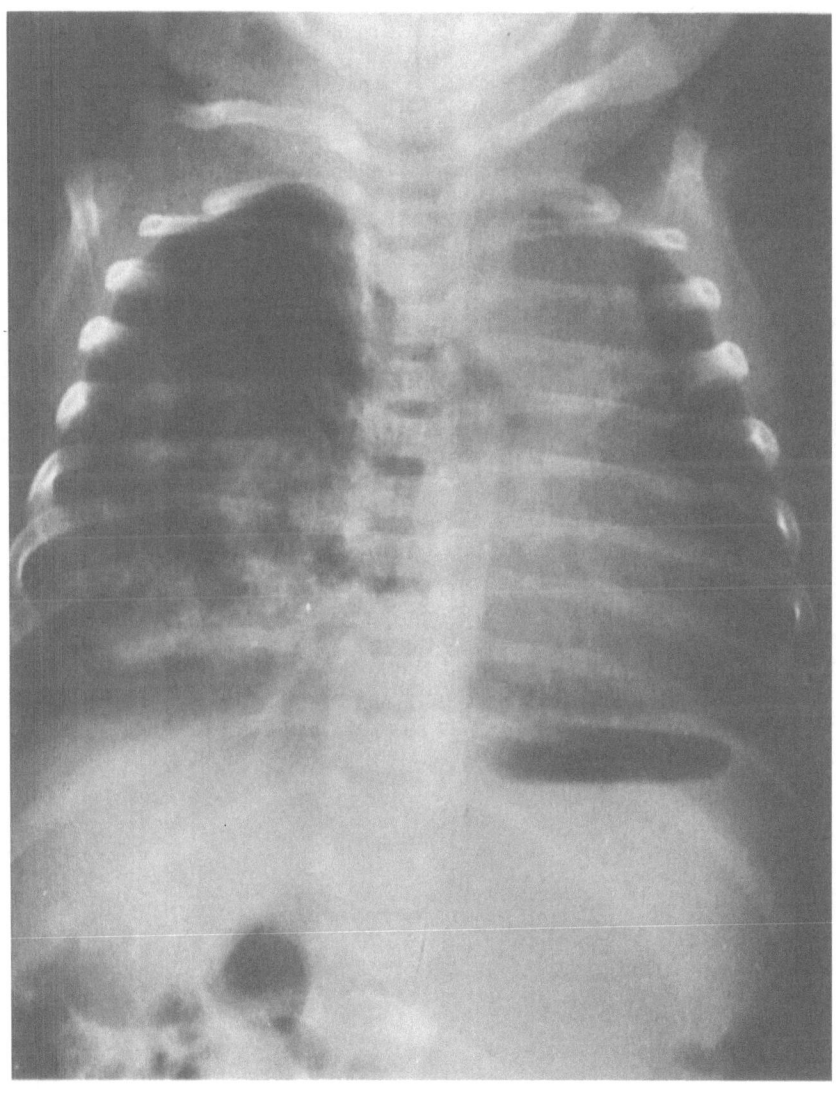

C37.1

Case 37. Answers:

1. a) The mediastinum is shifted to the left.
   b) Patchy shadowing is present in the right mid and lower zones.

2. The differential diagnosis should include: cystic adenomatous malformation of the lung (C37.2); infection (multiple small pneumatocoeles), but patient too young for this; right-sided diaphragmatic hernia (rare—but may occur following a streptococcal chest infection); sequestrated lung segment (final diagnosis).

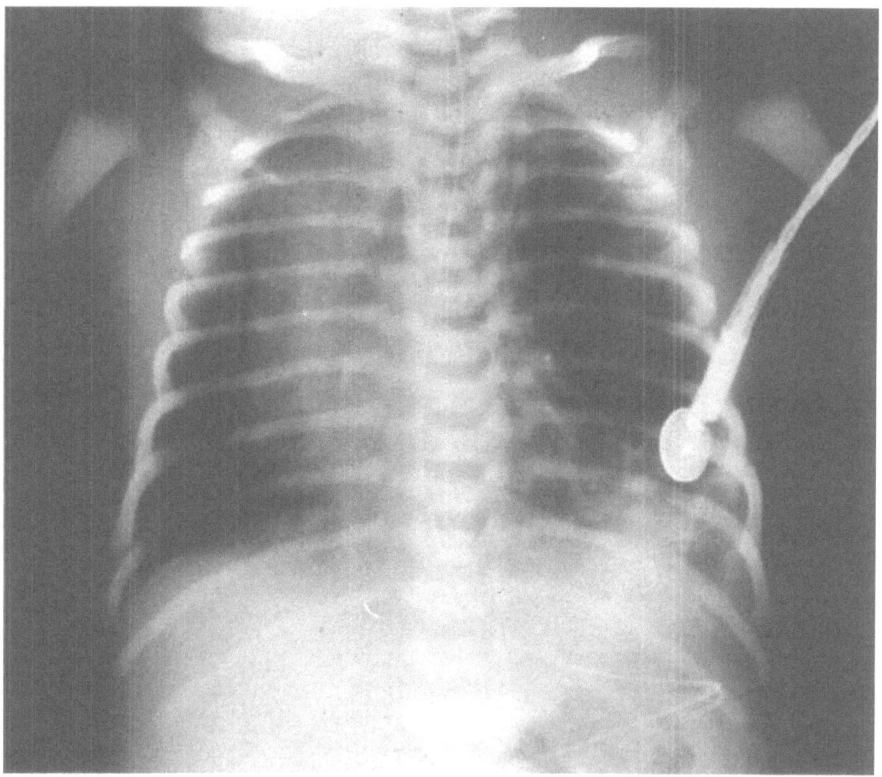

C37.2

Case 38. These are AP (C38.1) and lateral (C38.2) chest and abdominal radiographs in a 1-week-old neonate with marked respiratory distress.

Questions:

1. Describe two abnormalities in the chest.
2. What is the probable diagnosis?
3. What is the significance of the abdominal appearances?

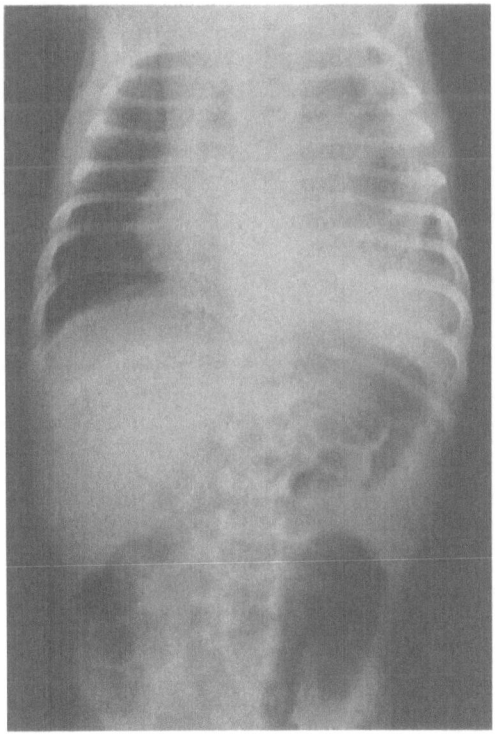

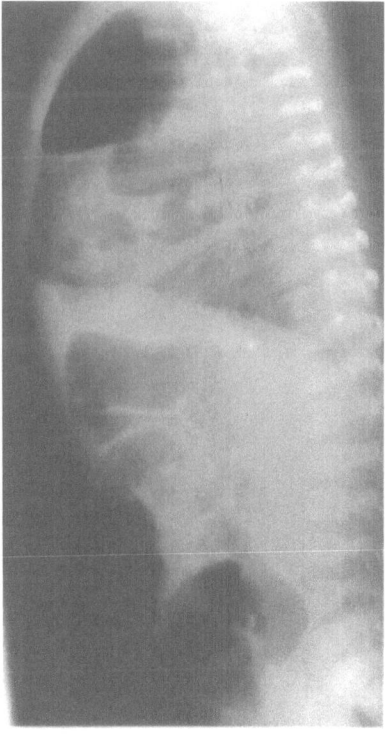

C38.1   C38.2

Case 38. Answers:

1. a) The mediastinum is deviated to the right.
   b) There are cystic areas with fluid levels in the left hemithorax (pneumato-coeles).

2. Staphylococcal pneumonia with pneumatocoeles.

3. This is not a Bochdalek-type of diaphragmatic hernia because of the normal bowel gas pattern in the abdomen.

Case 38. Comments:

Infected congenital lung cysts (which are very rare), a cystic adenomatous malformation of the lung or an infected sequestrated segment are other possible diagnoses. *E coli* pneumonia can produce similar pneumatocoeles.

Case 39. This full-term neonate presented within 2 h of birth with respiratory distress. A nasogastric tube and endotracheal tube were passed.

Questions:

1. Describe three major abnormalities on the chest and abdominal radiograph (C39.1).
2. What is the diagnosis?

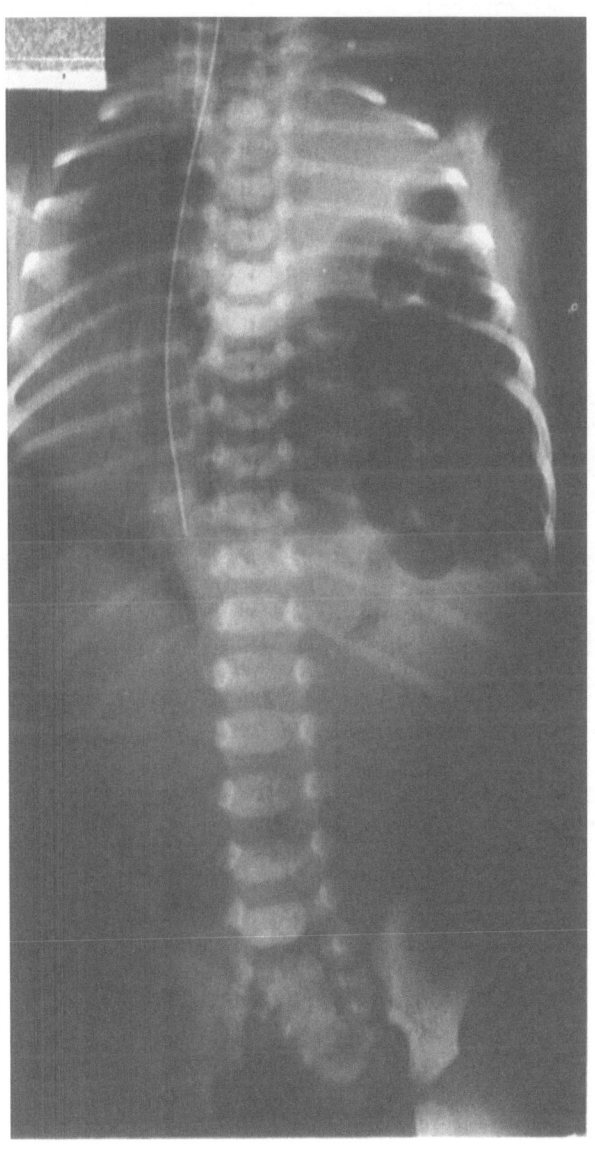

C39.1

Case 39. Answers:

1. a) "Cystic" appearance due to bowel gas in the left hemithorax.
   b) Mediastinal shift to the right.
   c) Absent bowel gas shadows in the abdomen.
2. Congenital diaphragmatic hernia (Bochdalek-type).

Case 39. Comments:

In many of these patients there is residual-lung hypoplasia on the left (C39.2).

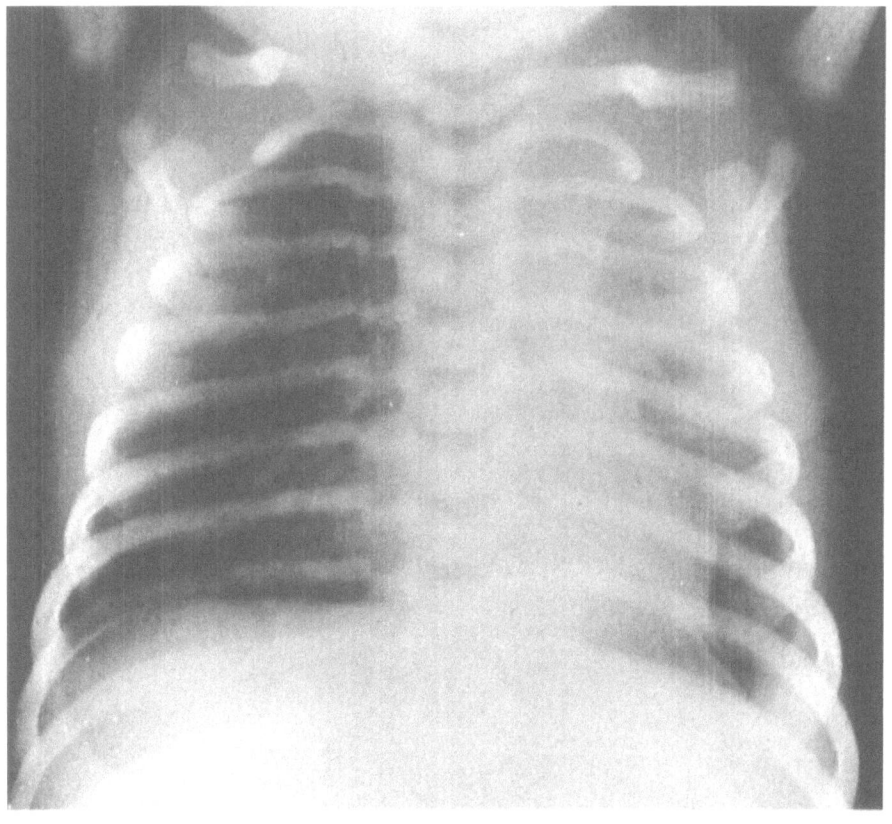

C39.2

Case 40. This 1-week-old neonate presented with respiratory distress.

Questions:

1. Describe the findings on the chest radiograph (C40.1).
2. What is the diagnosis?

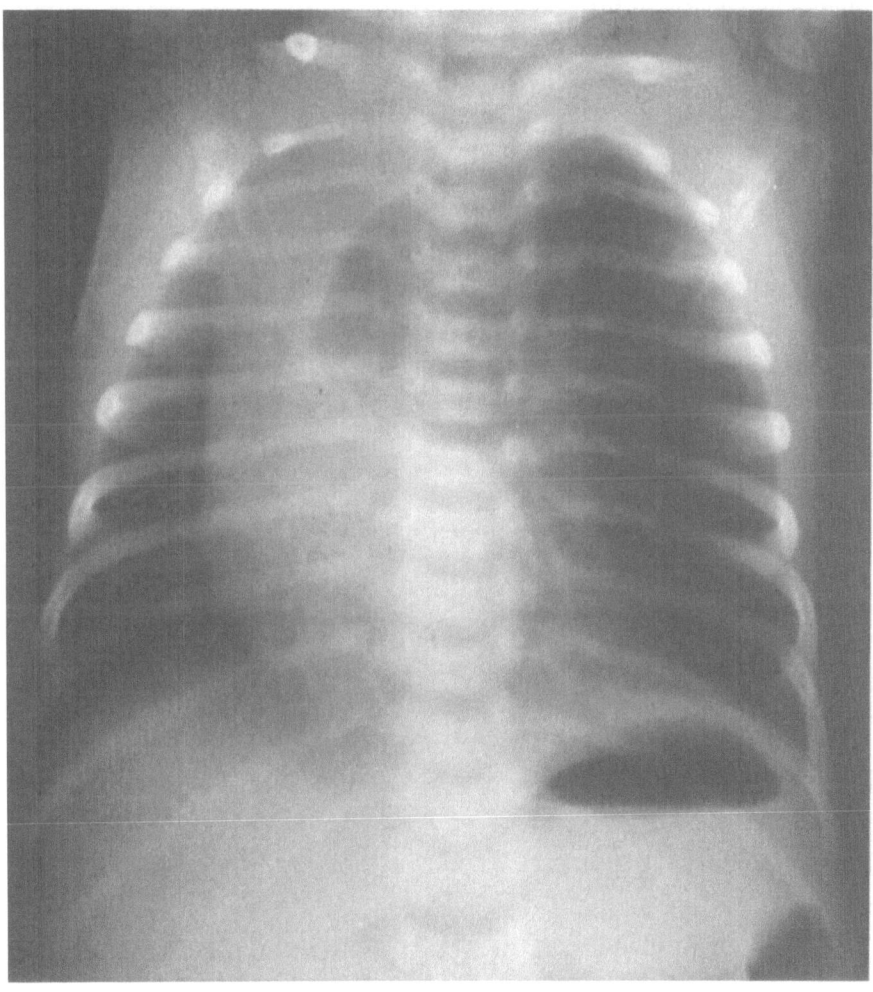

C40.1

Case 40. Answers:

1. There is mediastinal shift to the right caused by over-inflation on the left.
2. Congenital lobar emphysema.

Case 40. Comments:

The left upper lobe is most commonly affected in congenital lobar emphysema. There is air-trapping as a result of a congenital abnormality of the bronchial wall. The upper lobe may expand so much that it appears to involve the whole lung. Other cause of unilateral over-inflation of a lung/lobe include duplication/ neurenteric cyst, cystic adenomatous malformation, acquired cysts—pneumato-coeles, sequestrated segment, inhaled foreign body, compensatory emphysema (collapse/hypoplasia of the opposite lung) and bronchogenic cyst (as illustrated by C40.2). This left-sided bronchogenic cyst is causing air-trapping and over-inflation of the left upper lobe and collapse of the left lower lobe.

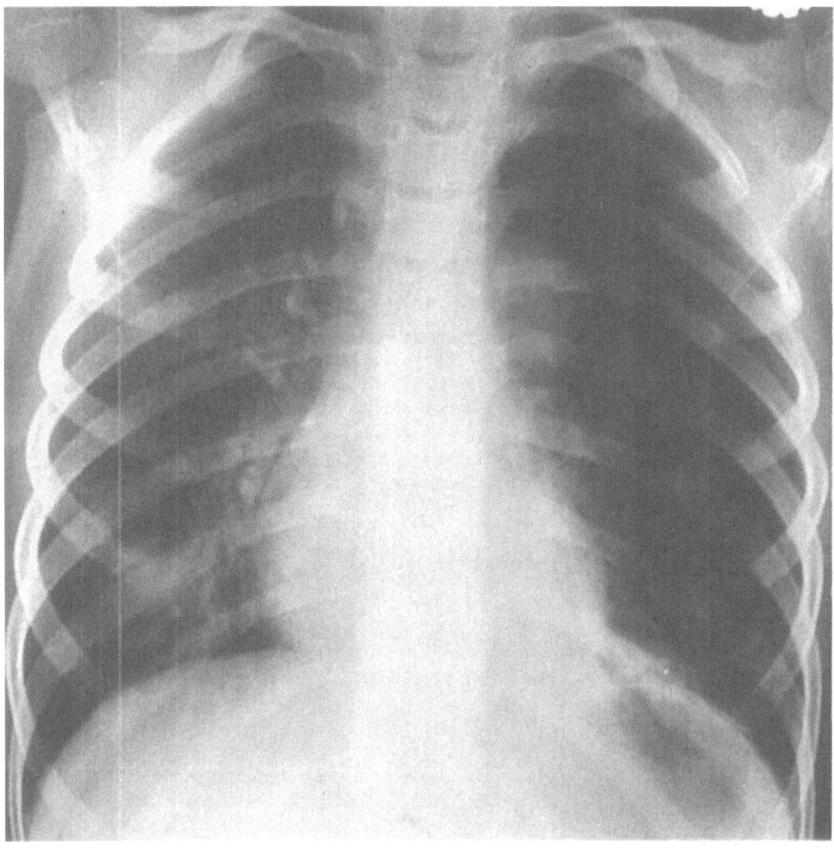

C40.2

Case 41.   This 6-week-old infant presented with wheeze and cough.

Questions:

1. What is the soft tissue opacity in the right upper zone (C41.1)?
2. Where is it on the lateral chest radiograph (C41.2)?
3. Name two other changes in the lung fields.

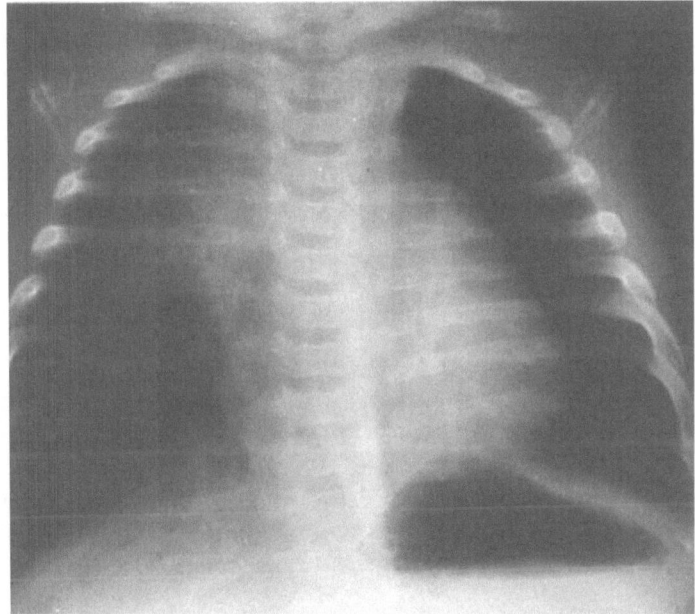

C41.1

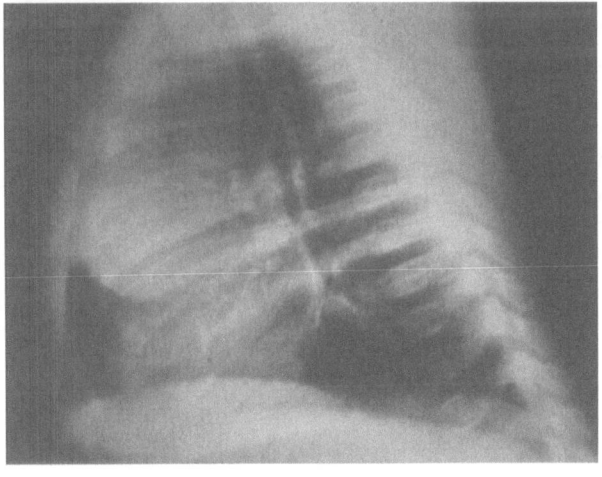

C41.2

Case 41. Answers:

1. Normal thymus.

2. Anterior mediastinum.

3. a) Over-inflation of the lungs causing flattening of the normal curve of the diaphgram.
   b) Streaky shadowing—caused by thickened bronchial walls—medially in the lung fields.

Case 41. Comments:

These two changes in an infant of this age are most likely a result of bronchiolitis: rarely a large but normal thymus may cause symptomatic tracheal compression.

Case 42. **This 4-month-old neonate presented with respiratory distress.**

Questions:

1. On this AP chest radiograph (C42.1) describe the abnormalities of the lung fields.

2. Describe any skeletal abnormalities.

3. What is the diagnosis?

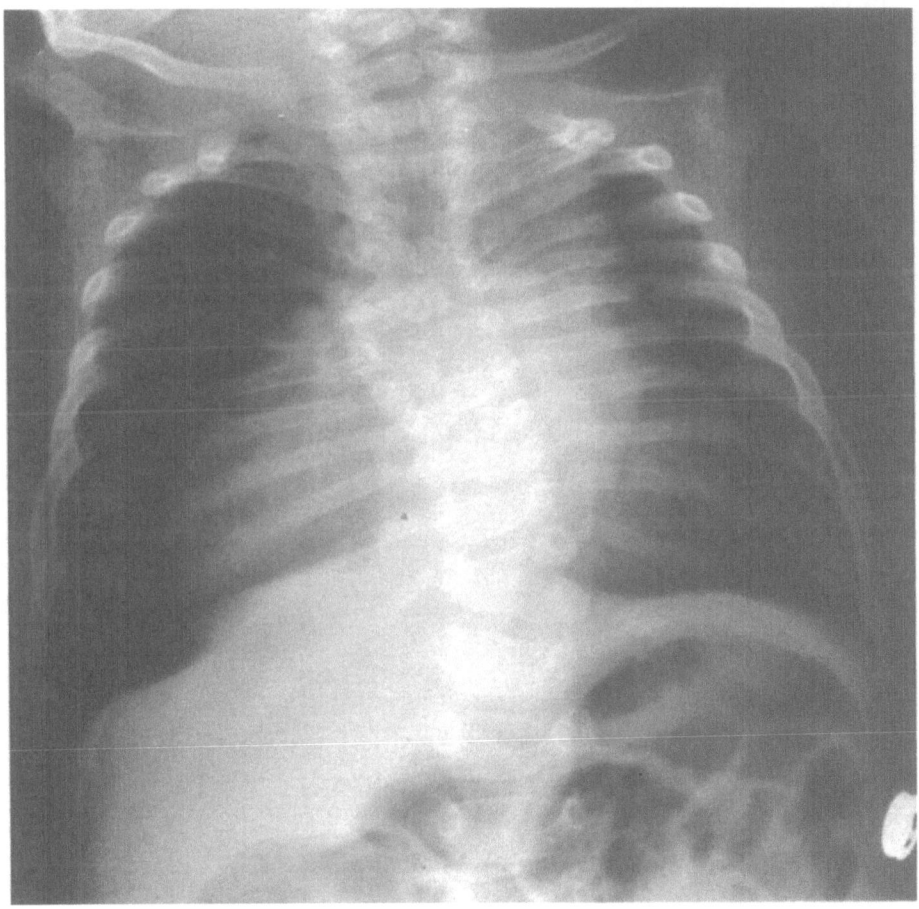

C42.1

Case 42. Answers:

1. There is a clearly defined rounded opacity of soft tissue density to the right of the midline and lying partially behind the heart. There is over-inflation with air-trapping in the right lower lobe, presumably caused by compression of the lower lobe bronchus.

2. There are right and left hemivertebrae with scoliosis, and anterior cleft vertebrae in the upper dorsal spine. Rib fusions are present.

3. Neurenteric duplication cyst.

Case 42. Comments:

The spinal anomalies indicate the potential communication of the cyst with the spinal canal (fibrous or communicating). These cysts usually contain some gastric mucosa and may present with a sudden bleed and acute respiratory distress.

Case 43. **This 8-month-old boy presented with a cough.**

Questions:

1. Describe the soft tissue abnormality on the chest radiograph (C43.1).
2. Describe the bony abnormalities.
3. Is the abnormality in the anterior, mid or posterior mediastinum?
4. What is the differential diagnosis?

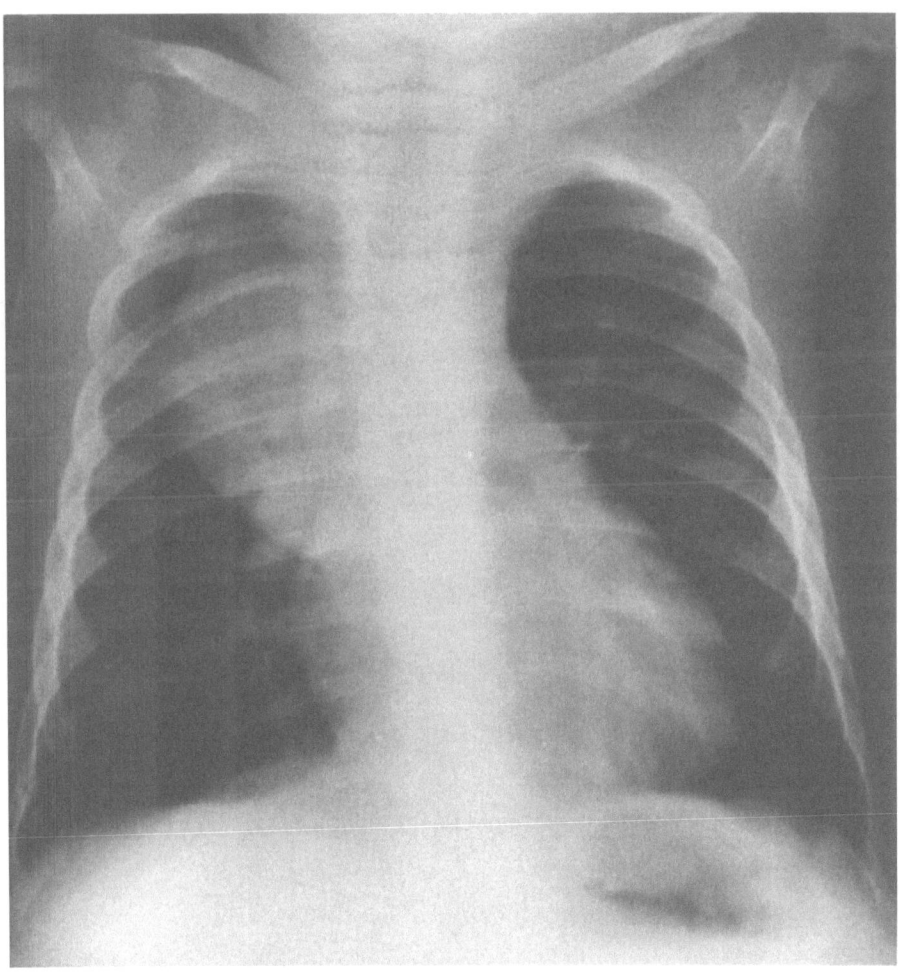

C43.1

Case 43. Answers:

1. There is a clearly defined, rounded mass adjacent to the right superior mediastinum.

2. There is splaying of the posterior ends of the second to fifth ribs with thinning of the fourth rib and inferior irregularity of the fourth and fifth ribs.

3. Posterior mediastinum.

4. Neurogenic tumour: ganglioneuroblastoma (benign or malignant), neuroblastoma (malignant) or neurofibromatosis.

Case 44. **This 2-year-old boy presented with stridor.**

Questions:

1. Describe the changes in the mediastinum (C44.1).
2. What other soft tissue abnormalities are present?
3. What is the diagnosis?

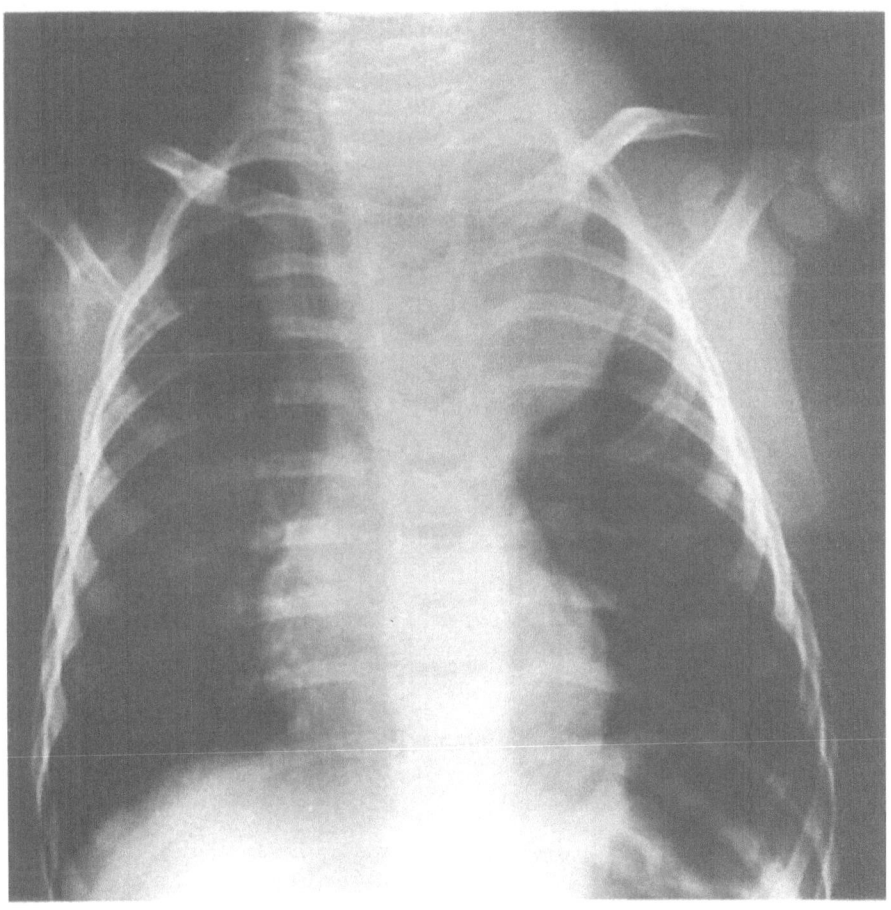

C44.1

Case 44. *Answers:*

1. There is a clearly defined soft tissue widening of the superior mediastinum, mainly to the left, causing displacement of the trachea to the right.

2. Soft tissue swelling is also present on the left side of the neck and in the left axilla.

3. Lymphoma. (Cystic hygroma should be considered, but extension into the axilla would not occur.)

Case 45. This 3-month-old boy was unwell with fever and tachypnoea. A follow-up chest radiograph (C45.2) was taken 1 week later.

Questions:

1. Describe the abnormalities on the original film (C45.1).
2. What were they due to?

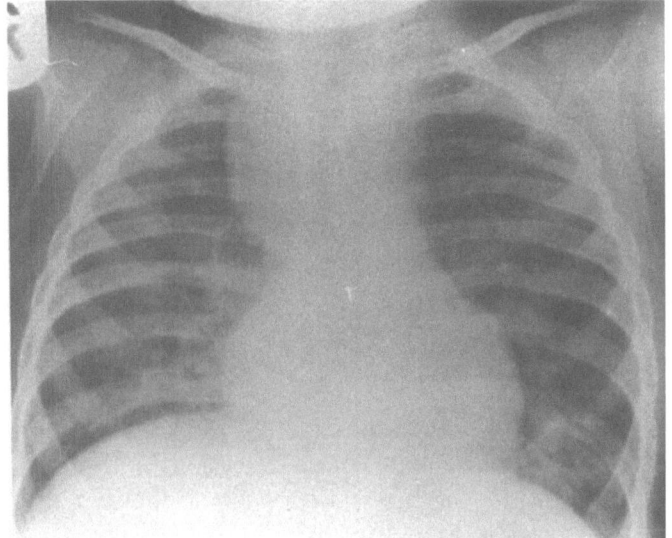

C45.1

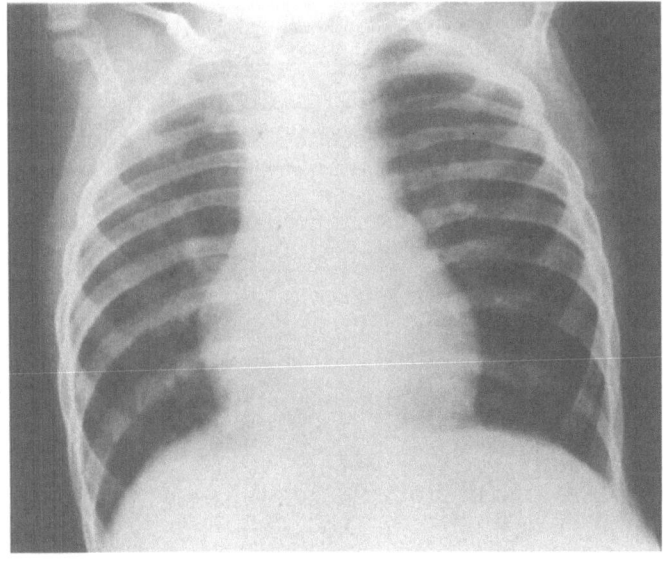

C45.2

Case 45. Answers:

1. There is widening of the superior mediastinum to the right with a clearly defined rounded lateral border. Patchy shadowing is present in both lower zones.

2. Consolidation with some collapse in an azygos lobe. The azygos fissure can be identified on the follow-up radiograph. There has also been considerable clearing of the basal consolidation. (Note the patient is rotated to the right.)

Case 46.   This is a chest radiograph (C46.1) of a 2-year-old child presenting with breathlessness.

Questions:

1. Describe two important findings.
2. What is the diagnosis?

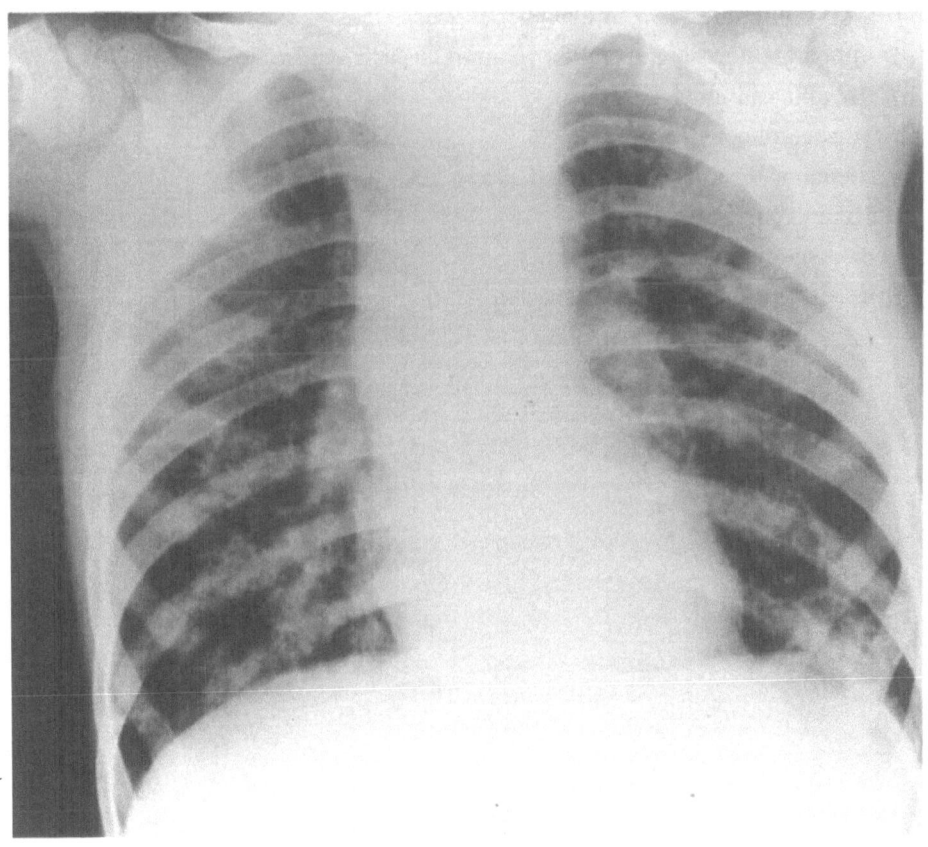

C46.1

Case 46. Answers:

1. a) "Honeycomb" appearance in both mid and lower zones.
   b) Clearly defined radiolucent area showing marginal sclerosis in the proximal right humeral shaft.
2. Eosinophilic granuloma (histiocystosis X).

Case 46. Comments:

Causes of a "honeycomb" appearance on a chest radiograph:

a) Histiocystosis X; Hand-Schüller-Christian disease, eosinophilic granuloma, Letterer-Siewe disease.
b) Tuberose sclerosis.
c) Cystic fibrosis (usually upper zone predominance).
d) Sarcoidosis.
e) Scleroderma.
f) Severe infantile form of Gaucher's disease.
g) Idiopathic fibrosing alveolitis (Hammon-Rich syndrome).
h) Rheumatoid lung.
i) Mucocutaneous candidiasis.
j) Niemann-Pick disease.
k) Mikety-Wilson syndrome.
l) Bronchopulmonary dysplasia.
m) Recurrent sensitivity pneumonitis.

Case 47. This 5-year-old girl presented with failure to thrive and cough and wheeze.

Questions:

1. Describe the abnormalities in the lung fields (C47.1).
2. What is the differential diagnosis?

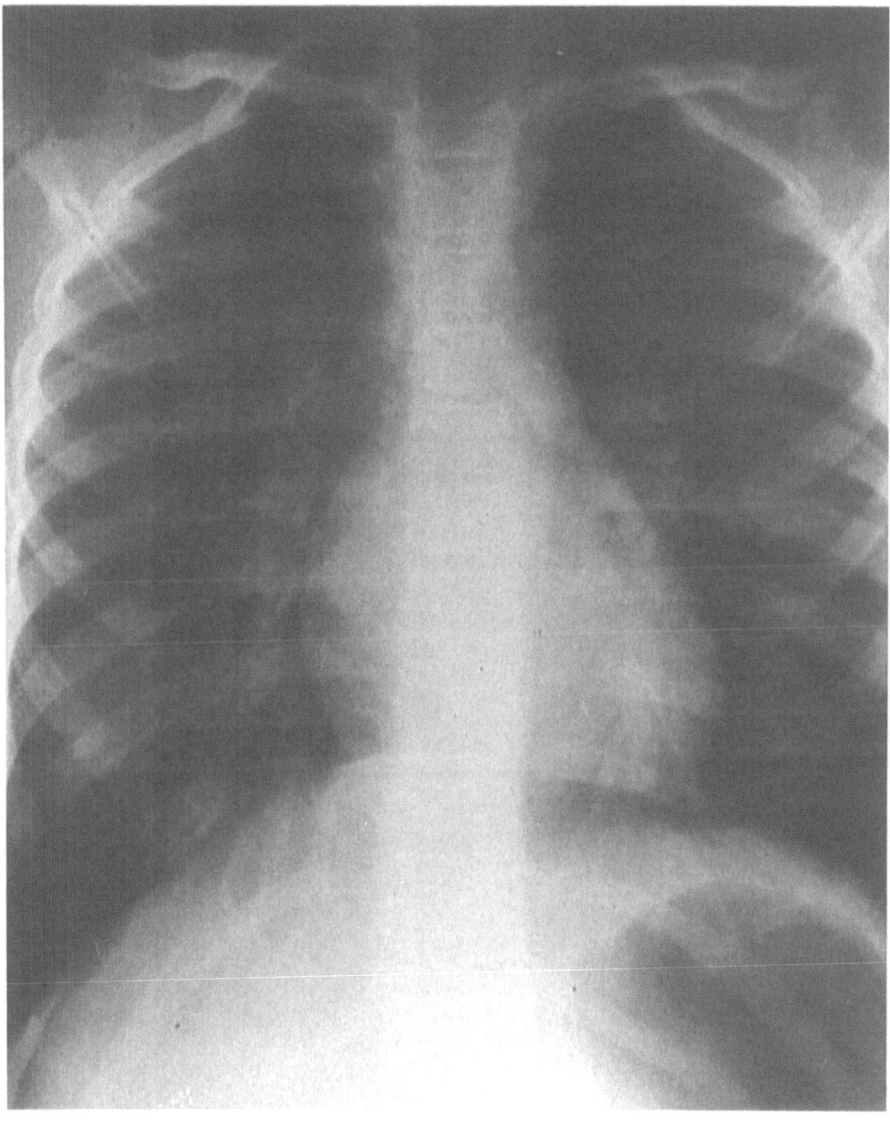

C47.1

Case 47. Answers:

1. a) Over-inflation (loss of normal diaphragmatic curve especially on the right).
   b) Generalised bronchial wall thickening giving rise to ring shadows, and parallel "tramline" shadows.
   c) Right lower zone consolidation.

2. In a child of this age the following should all be considered: cystic fibrosis (upper zone changes often predominate), asthma, whooping cough and chronic bronchitis.

Case 47. Comments:

This child has cystic fibrosis. The changes on the OM (occipito-mental) view of her sinuses are illustrated below (C47.2). Both maxillary antra and the right ethmoid and right frontal sinuses are opaque. This is a result of the generalised increased "stickiness" of secretions of the exocrine glands. This condition is also called mucoviscidosis.

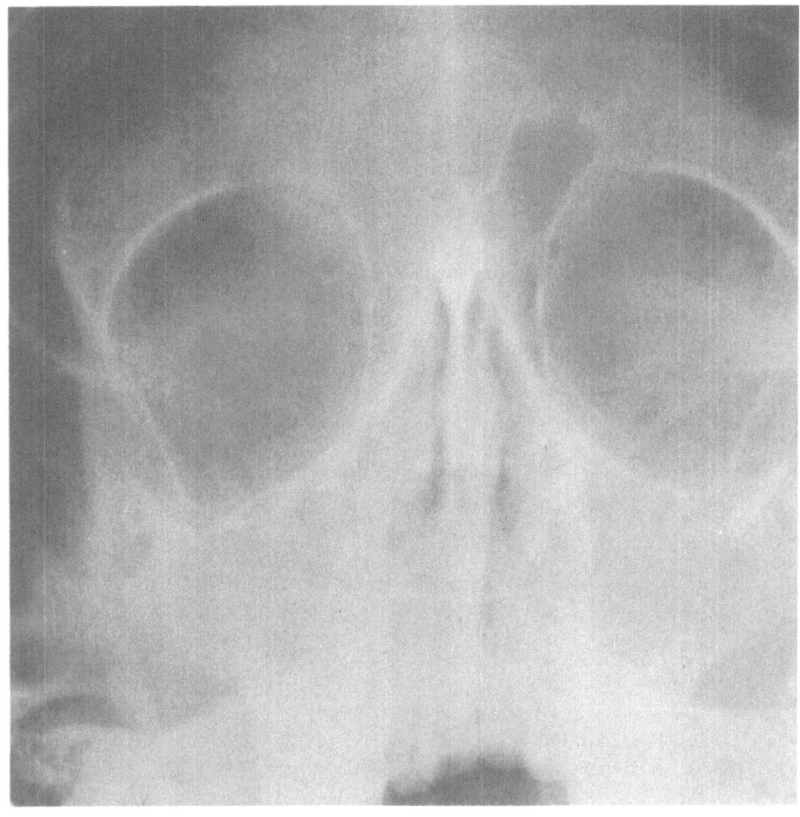

C47.2

Case 48. This 6-year-old boy presented with acute chest pain and respiratory distress. He was known to suffer from chronic lung disease.

Questions:

1. Describe two major abnormalities of the lung fields (C48.1).
2. What is the differential diagnosis?

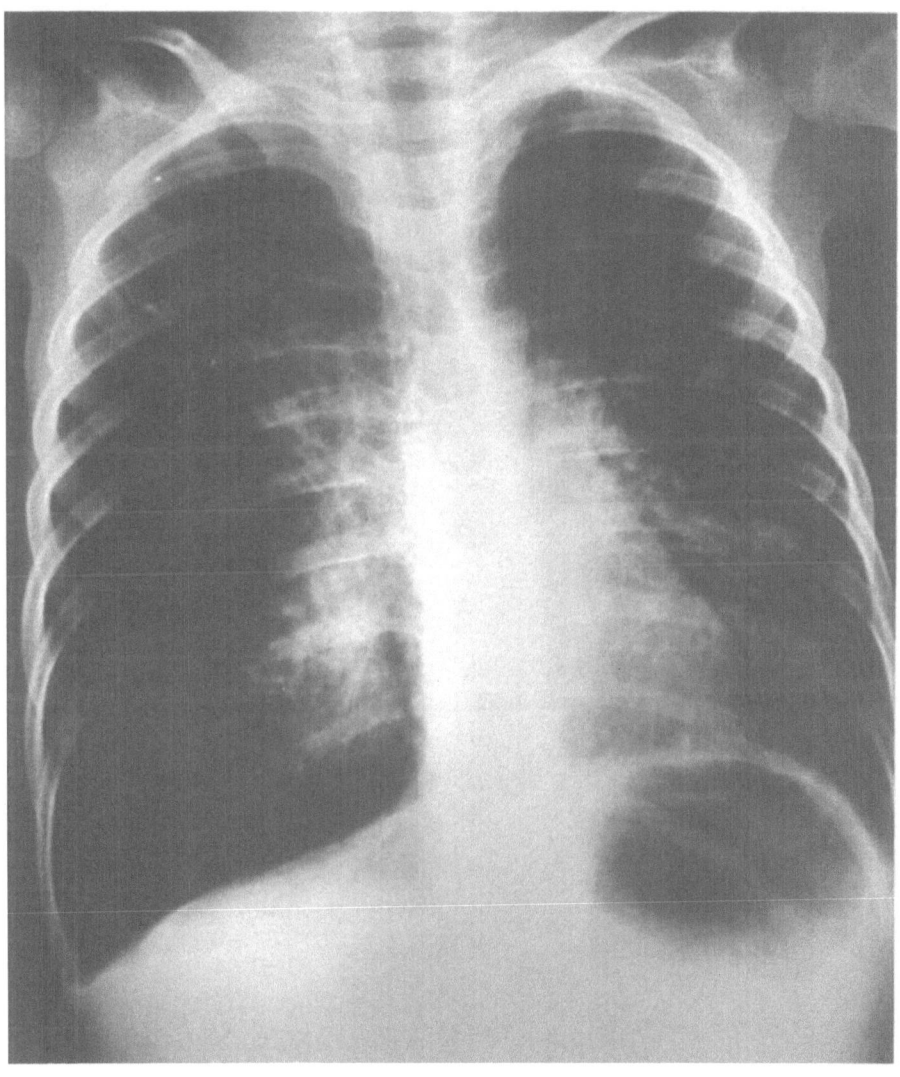

C48.1

Case 48. Answers:

1. a) Right-sided pneumothorax.
   b) Honeycomb lung.
2. The differential diagnosis of a honeycomb lung is shown on p. 92. This child had idiopathic fibrosing alveolitis.

Case 48. Comments:

C48.2 illustrates a left-sided pneumothorax in a child with cystic fibrosis.

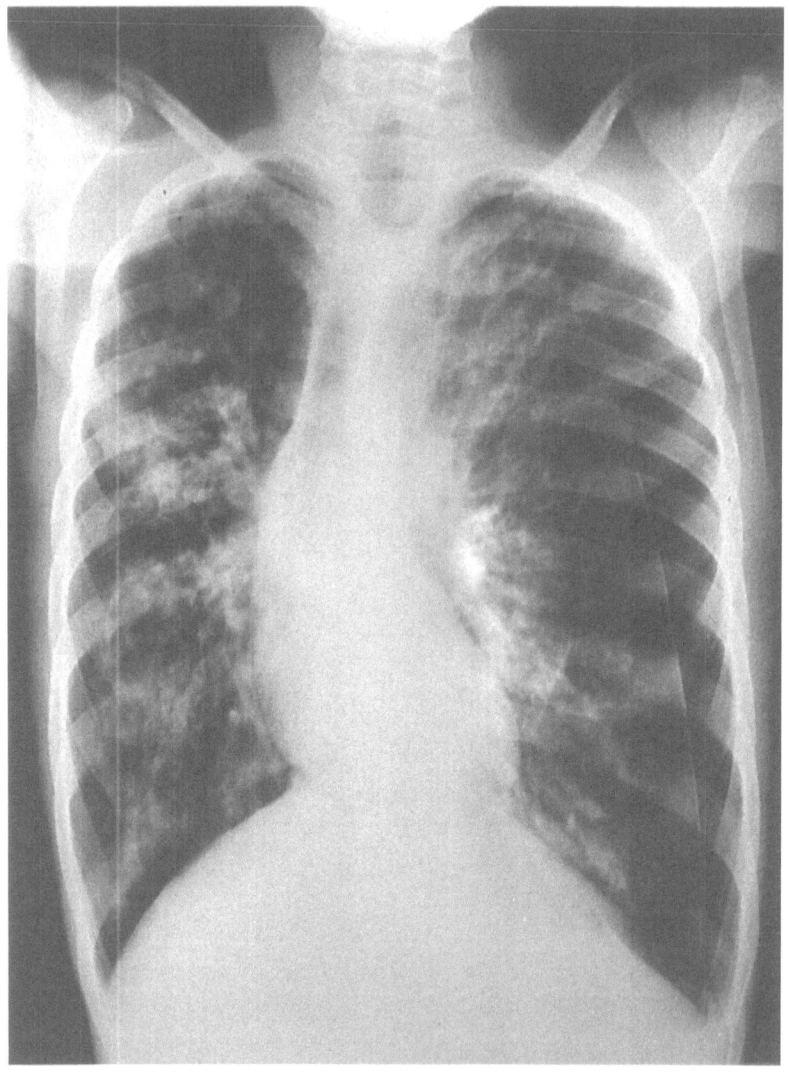

C48.2

Case 49.   This 6-year-old girl has had recurrent chest infections.

Questions:

1. Describe the abnormalities on the chest radiograph (C49.1).
2. What is the differential diagnosis?

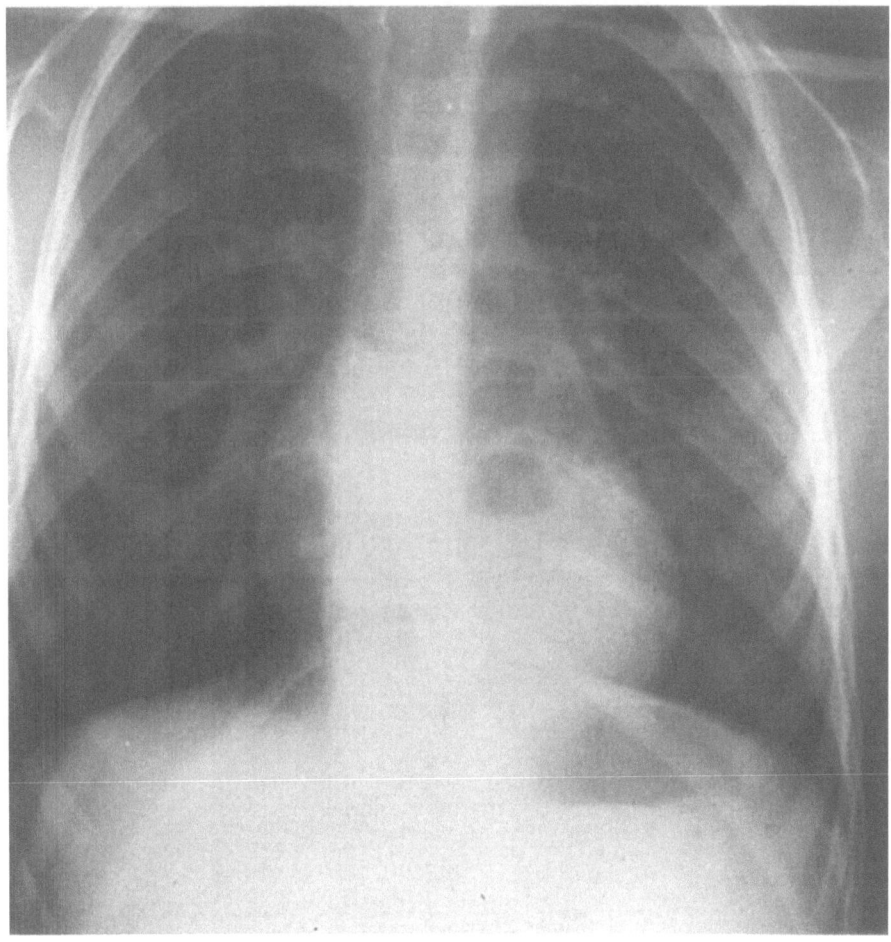

C49.1

Case 49. Answers:

1. There is a double density behind the heart shadow with an air-fluid level.

2. a) Pneumonia with abscess formation.
   b) Hiatus hernia.
   c) Infected sequestrated segment (final diagnosis).
   d) Infected lung cyst/pneumatocoele.

Case 49. Comments:

The flush aortic angiogram (C49.2) demonstrates the arterial supply to the sequestrated lung segment. This is arising from below the diaphragm. The air/fluid level indicates not only the presence of infection, but communication with the bronchial tree.

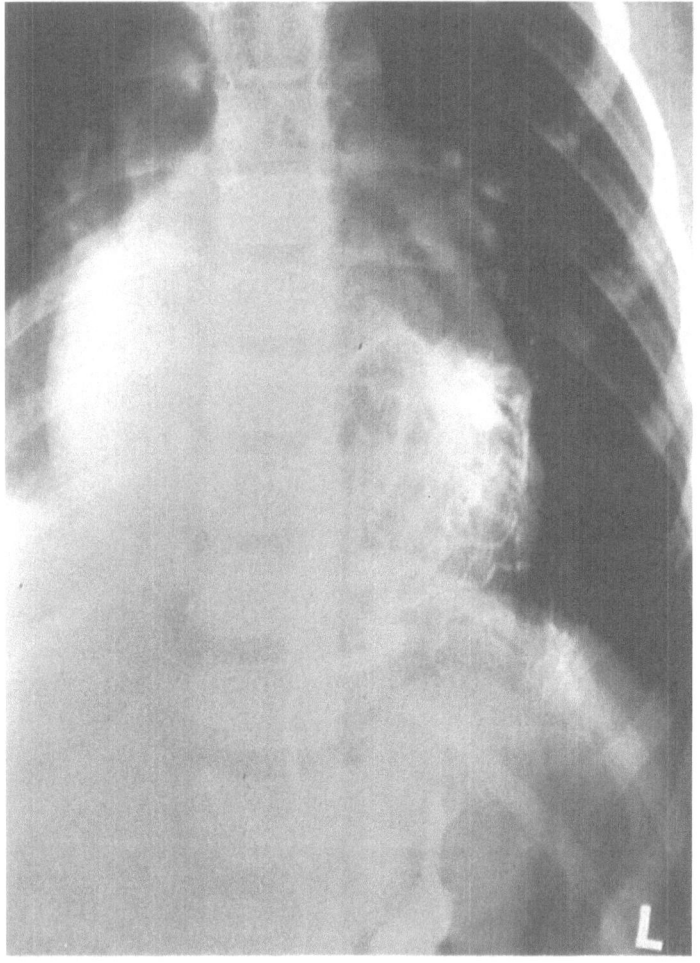

C49.2

Case 50. This 10-year-old boy presented with recurrent chest infections.

Questions:

1. Describe four major abnormalities on the chest radiograph (C50.1).
2. What is the name of the condition?
3. What is it caused by?

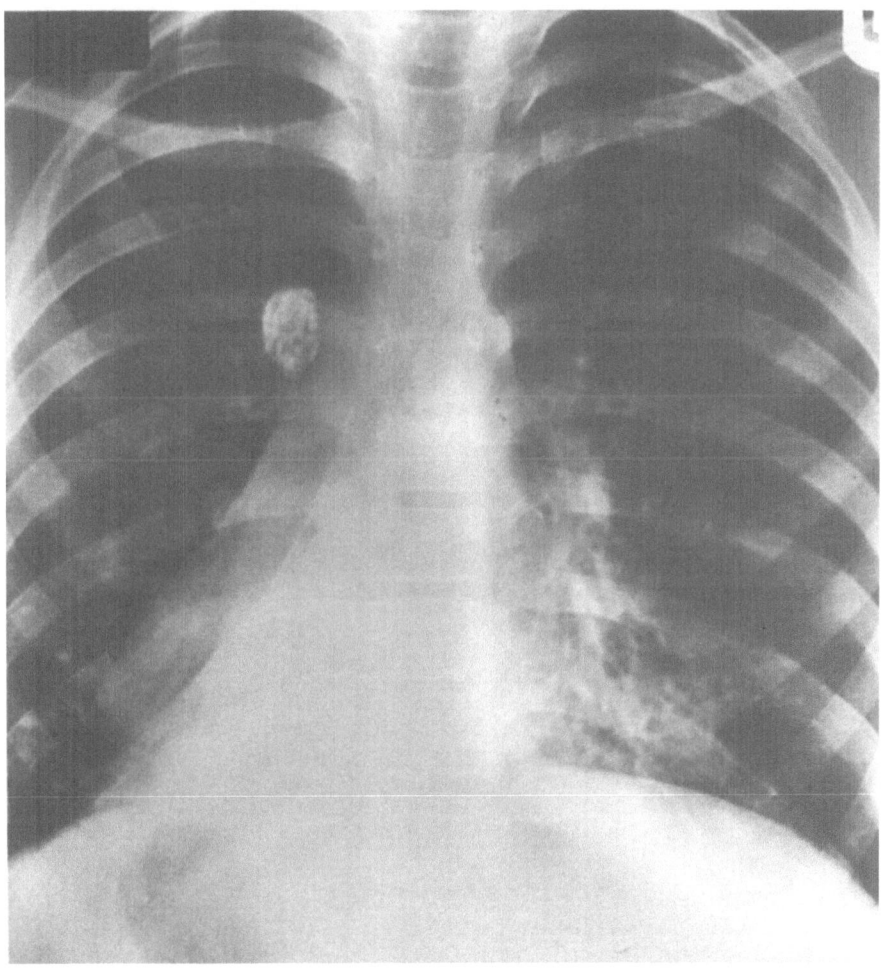

C50.1

Case 50. *Answers:*

1. a) Total situs inversus.
   b) Collapse of the right lower lobe and mediastinal shift to the right.
   c) Bronchial wall thickening due to bronchiectasis in the left lower lobe.
   d) Calcified right hilar gland due to old tuberculosis.

2. Kartagener's syndrome.

3. Decreased ciliary motility.

Case 51. This 3-month-old infant has had episodes of heart failure and chest infections.

Questions:

1. Describe a mediastinal abnormality (C51.1).
2. What is wrong with the right lung?
3. What is the "band" shadowing at the right base due to?
4. What is this condition and what is the name of the syndrome?

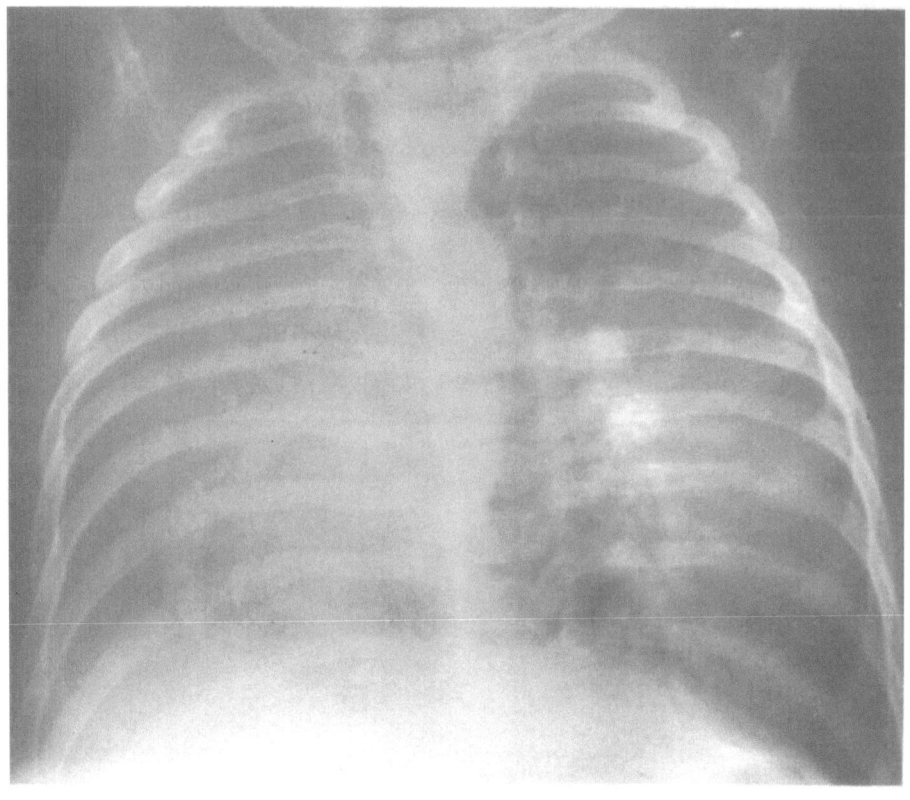

C51.1

Case 51. Answers:

1. Mediastinum shifted to the right.
2. Hypoplastic right lung.
3. Anomalous veins passing through the diaphragm.
4. Partial anomalous pulmonary venous drainage. Scimitar syndrome.

Case 51. Comments:

Other conditions associated with unilateral congenital lung hypoplasia include:

a) VATER association (C51.2)—renal, vertebral and oesophageal atresia changes are illustrated.

b) Oesophageal lung (C51.3) post anastomotic study for oesophageal atresia. The right main bronchus arises from the lower oesophagus.

c) Diaphragmatic hernia.

d) Accessory diaphragm.

e) Pulmonary artery hypoplasia/aplasia.

f) Tetralogy of Fallot.

g) Truncus arteriosus.

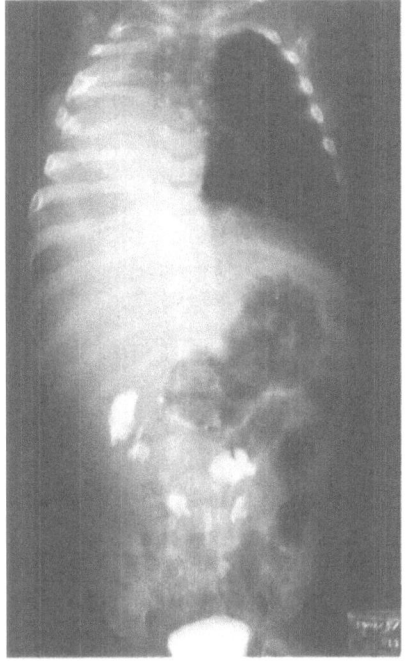

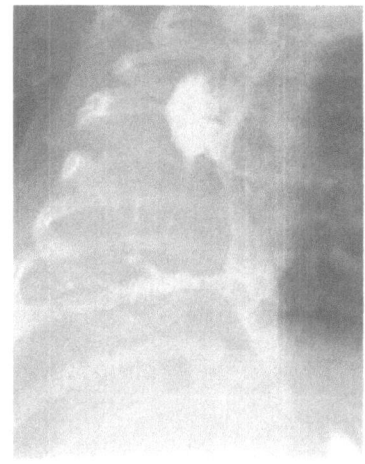

C51.2   C51.3

Case 52. **This 8-year-old girl presented with a respiratory tract infection.**

Questions:

1. Describe the changes on the AP chest radiograph (C52.1).
2. What are the changes due to?
3. On the lateral radiograph (C52.2), which dome of the diaphragm corresponds to which side? Give three reasons.

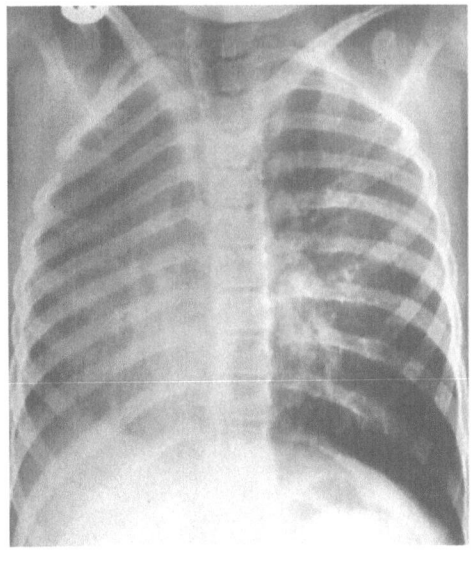

C52.1

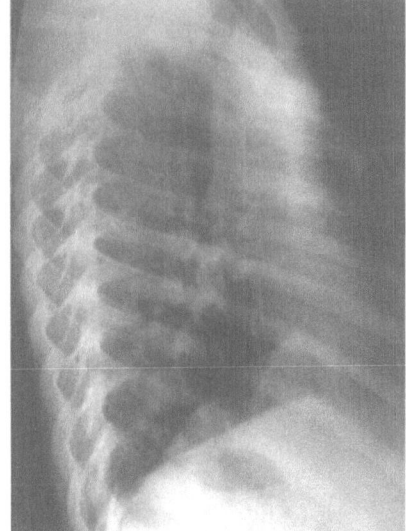

C52.2

Case 52. Answers:

1. There is mediastinal shift to the right. Hazy opacification is present over the right hemithorax. Increased prominence of vascular markings on the left is present (due to increased pulmonary blood flow through the left lung).

2. Hypoplasia of the right lung.

3. The higher dome is on the right side.
   a) Reduced lung volume on right causes elevation of right dome.
   b) Air bubble in the fundus of the stomach is adjacent to the left dome (lower dome).
   c) The left dome terminates anteriorly at the junction with the cardiac border. This is slightly more anterior than usual due to the mediastinal shift to the right.

Case 53.   **This 6-year-old child with asthma presented with fever.**

Questions:

1. Describe the abnormalities in the lung fields on this lateral chest radiograph (C53.1).

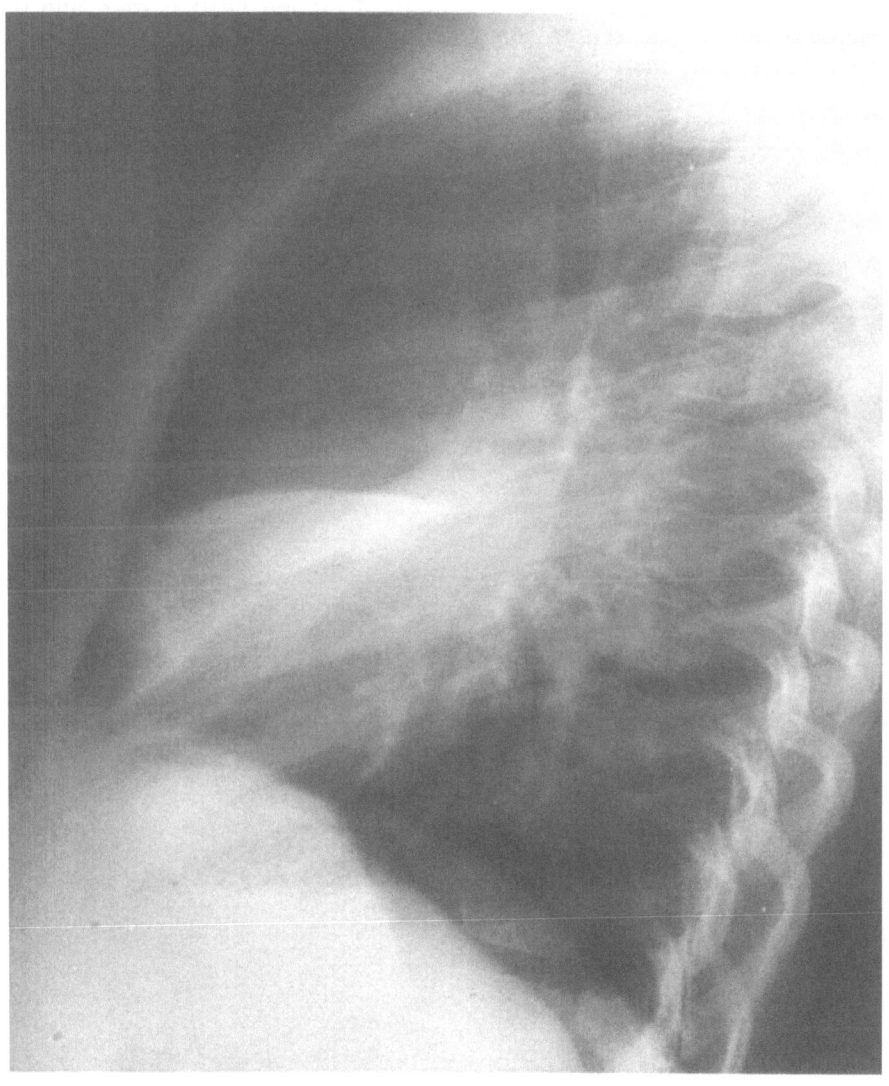

C53.1

Case 53. Answers:

1. There is collapse and consolidation in the middle lobe and lingula. (There is evidence of consolidation adjacent to both oblique fissures.) There is some over-inflation with flattening of the diaphragm, and bronchial wall shadowing is evident in the lower lobes.

Case 53. Comments:

The AP chest radiograph (C53.2) confirms these findings. The lingular consolidation gives rise to loss of definition of the left heart border, and the collapse on the left has caused depression of the left hilar point (normally it is higher than that on the right).

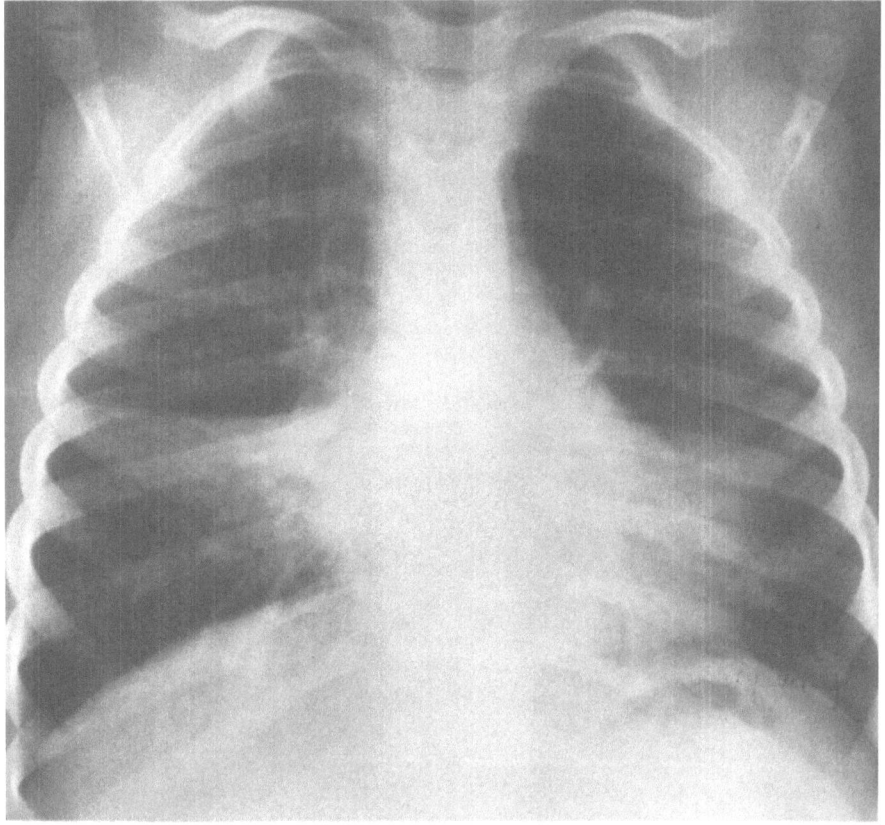

C53.2

Case 54. This 8-month-old child presented with a cough.

Questions:

1. Describe four significant abnormalities on the AP view of the chest (C54.1).
2. What further investigation would you request?
3. What is the possible diagnosis?

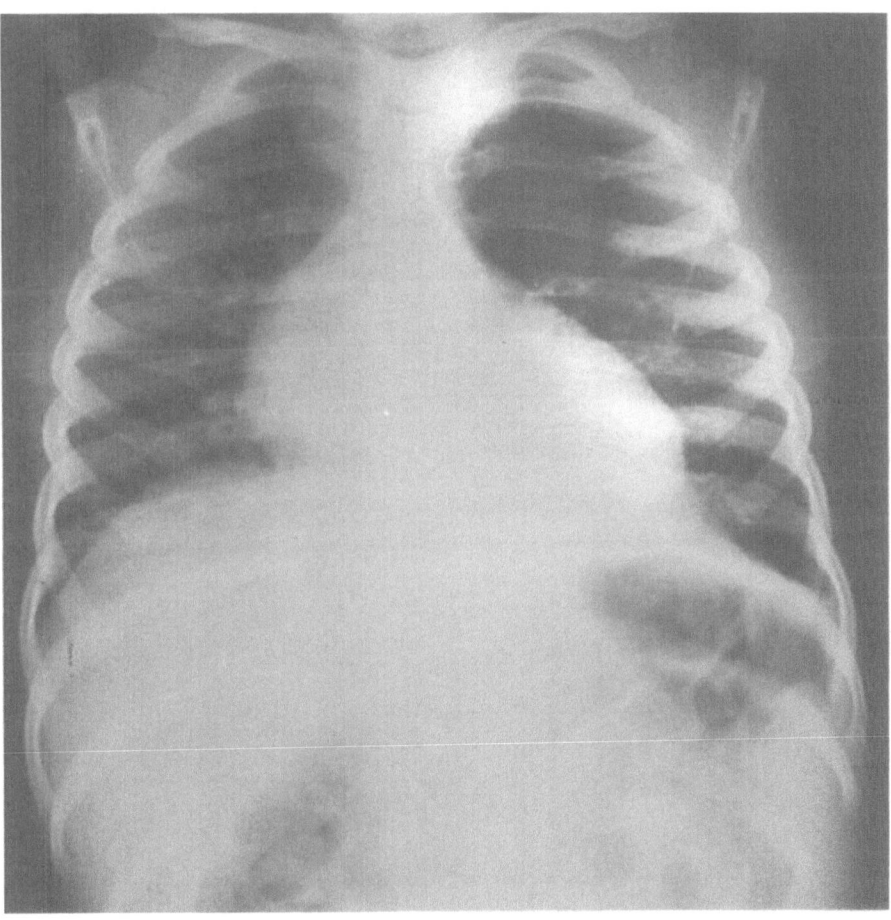

C54.1

Case 54. *Answers:*

1. a) Mediastinal shift to the right.
   b) Over-inflation of the left upper lobe.
   c) Collapse of the left lower lobe.
   d) Low left dome of diaphragm.

2. Screening of the diaphragm (to assess for air-trapping—the left diaphragm remains low on expiration and the mediastinum swings further to the right). Note: expiratory films may be difficult to obtain at this age.

3. Inhaled foreign body in the left main bronchus with occlusion of the left lower lobe bronchus and collapse; ball-valve obstruction of the left upper lobe bronchus with air-trapping.

Case 55. This 3-year-old Indian boy had been unwell for several weeks.

Questions:

1. Describe the abnormalities on the chest radiograph (C55.1).
2. What is the likely diagnosis?
3. What other radiographic abnormalities in the chest are likely in this condition?

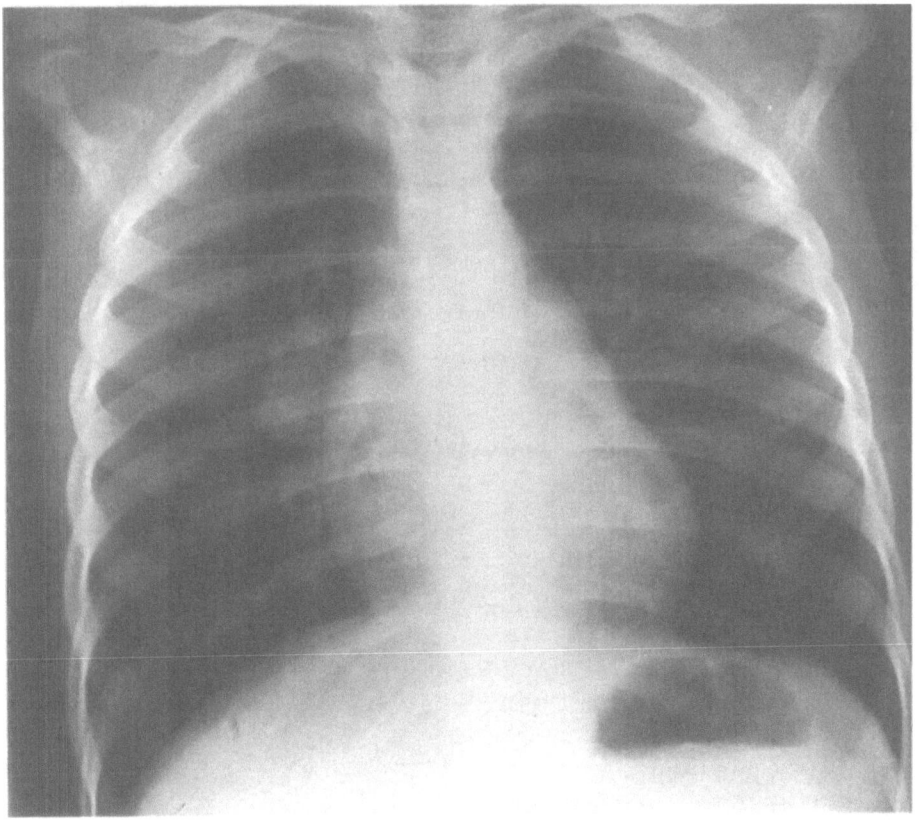

C55.1

Case 55. Answers:

1. There is right-sided hilar gland enlargement.

2. Tuberculosis.

3. Diffuse miliary shadowing (C55.2); segmental collapse; apical contraction and calcification (C55.3); endobronchial granulomata with collapse (C55.4); pleural effusion/thickening; paraspinal shadowing with spinal involvement.

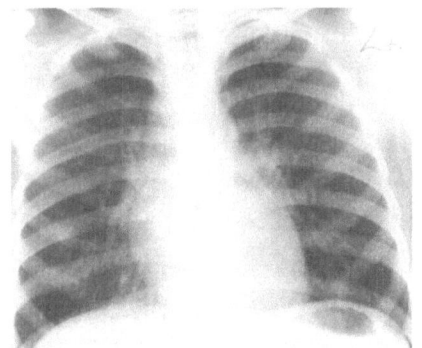

C55.2

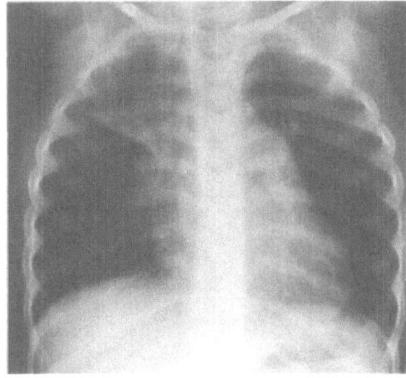

C55.3

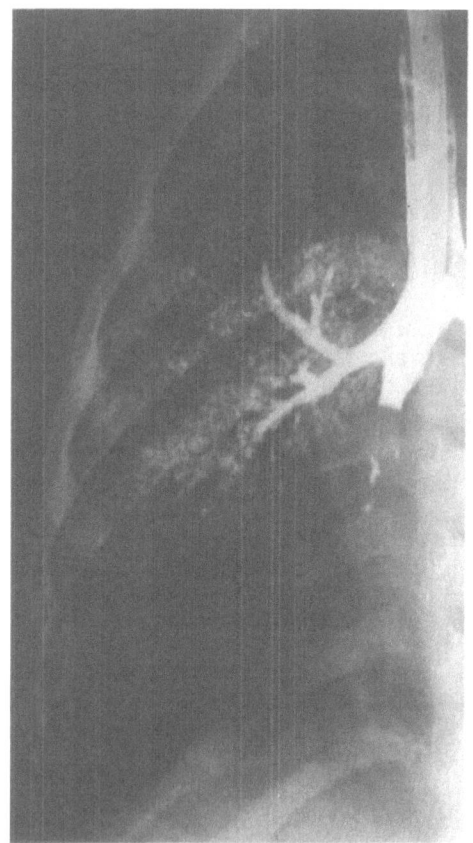

C55.4

Case 56. This 4-year-old boy had been followed for a cardiac problem since infancy. He had recently started school and tired easily. On examination he had a pan-systolic murmur.

Questions:

1. Describe the abnormalities on the AP chest radiograph (C56.1).

2. What is the diagnosis?

3. List the signs of heart failure which you would expect to see on a chest radiograph.

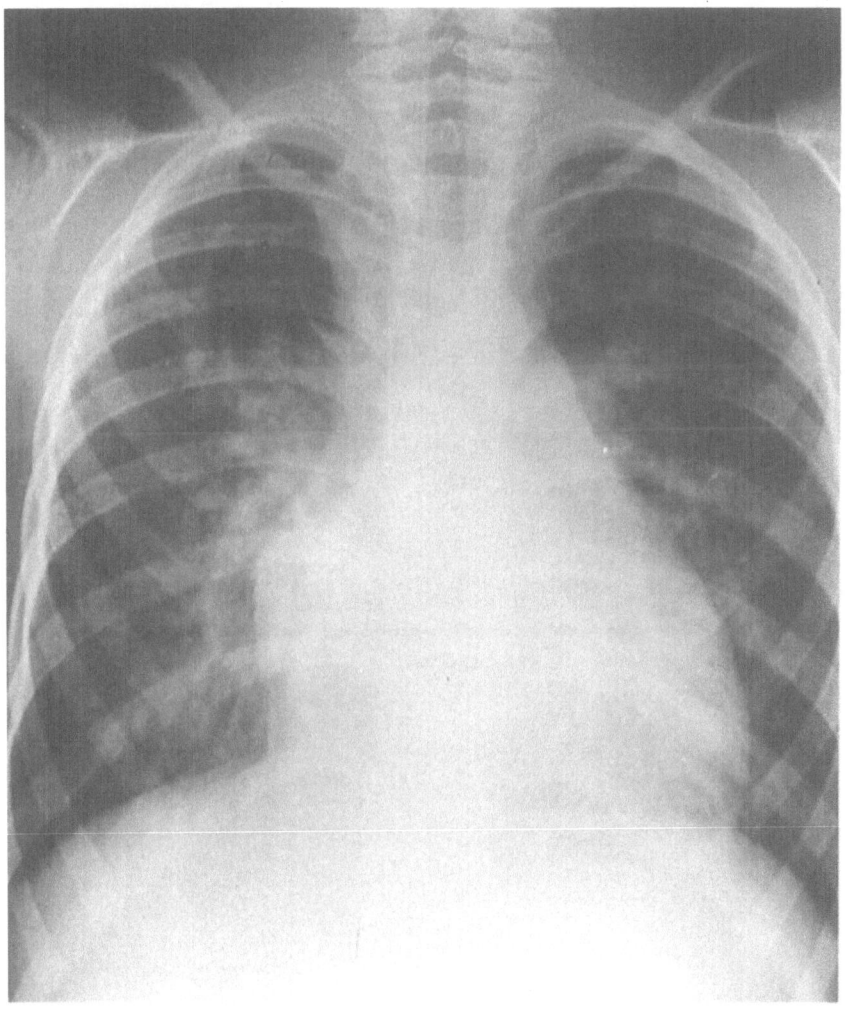

C56.1

Case 56. Answers:

1. The heart is enlarged and the lung fields plethoric but otherwise clear. Some left atrial enlargement. An azygos lobe is present.

2. Ventricular septal defect.

3. Cardiac enlargement—especially left ventricle and left atrium; upper zone blood diversion; perivascular cuffing; pulmonary oedema—initially perihilar; pleural effusions with filling-in of the costophrenic angles and fluid in the horizontal fissure; septal b-lines at the bases; liver enlargement.

Case 56. Comments:

C56.2 illustrates some of the features of heart failure in the same boy 4 days after repair of the ventricular septal defect.

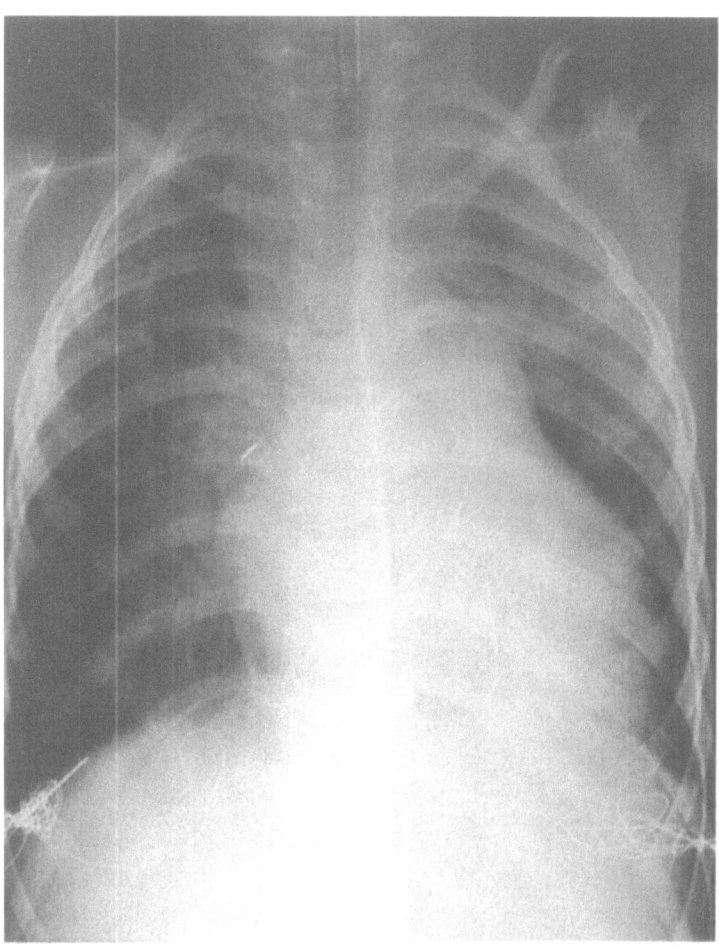

C56.2

Case 57. This 9-month-old boy had been cyanosed since birth. He had just undergone surgery, as evidenced by the left-sided pleural effusion and the soft tissue swelling at the angle of the left scapula.

Questions:

1. Is the heart enlarged (C57.1)?
2. Describe the abnormality of the left cardiac border. What does it indicate?
3. Are the lung fields plethoric or oligaemic?
4. What is the likely diagnosis?
5. What was the nature of the surgery and why was it performed on the left?

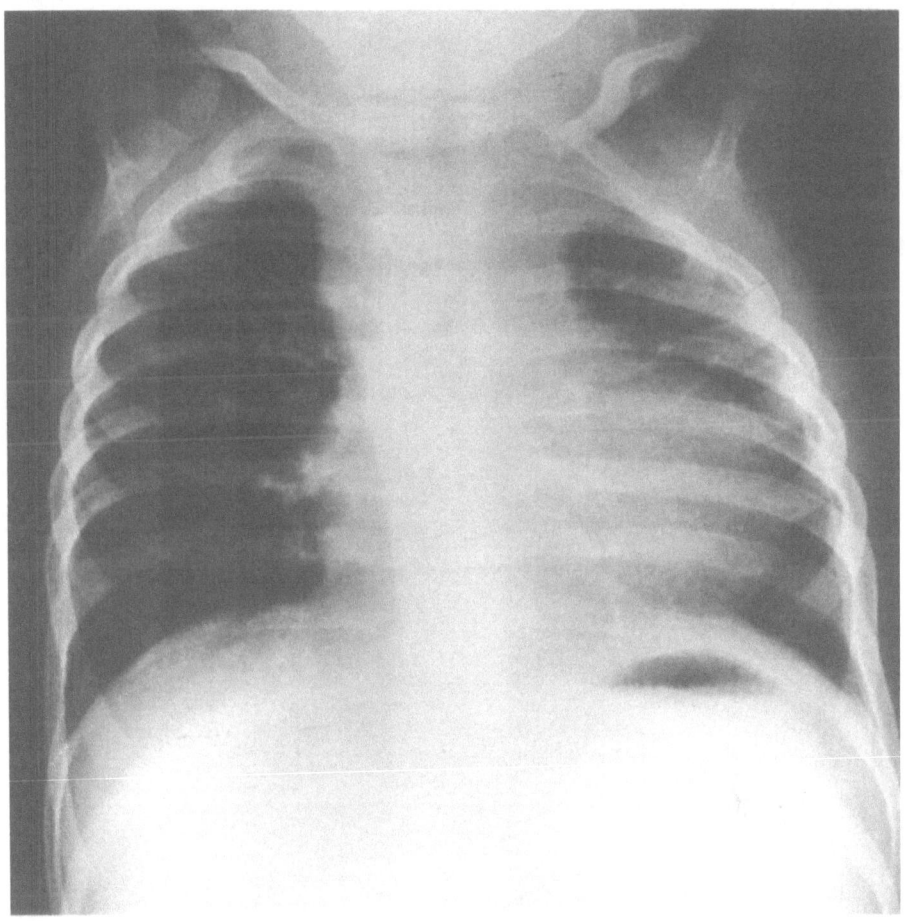

C57.1

113

Case 57. *Answers:*

1. Yes.

2. Deep pulmonary bay and high apex of heart. The deep pulmonary bay indicates a small pulmonary outflow tract. The high apex indicates predominant right ventricular enlargement.

3. The lung fields are oligaemic.

4. Fallot situation (including pulmonary atresia).

5. A Blalock-Taussig shunt was performed on the left because there is a right-sided aortic arch.

Case 57. *Comments:*

Other conditions associated with a right-sided aortic arch when the cardiac apex is on the left:

a) truncus arteriosus.

b) Fallot situation (including pulmonary atresia).

c) Uncomplicated ventricular septal defect.

d) vascular ring.

Case 58. This 5-week-old infant has had stridor since birth.

Questions:

1. Describe two significant findings on this lateral view of a barium swallow (C58.1).
2. What is the cause of the stridor?

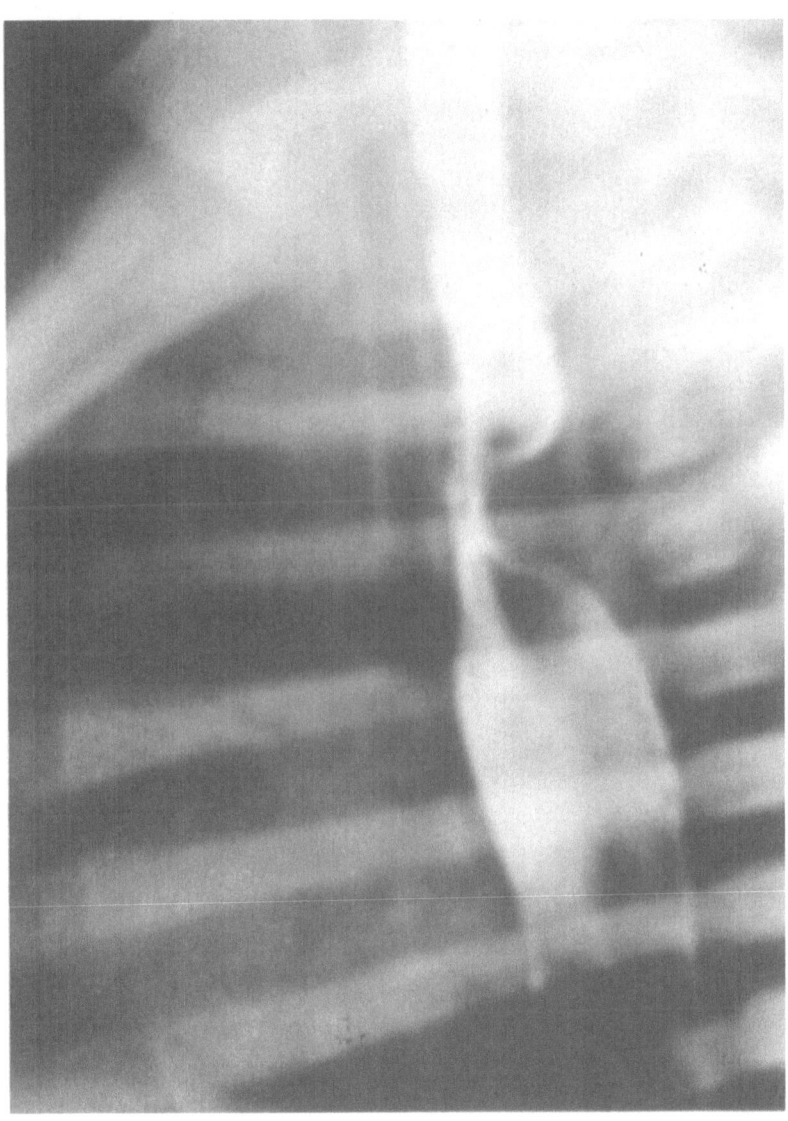

C58.1

Case 58. Answers:

1. a) An extrinsic posterior impression on the oesophagus.
   b) An endotracheal tube.
2. Vascular ring.

Case 58. Comments:

The endotracheal tube must be long enough to be below the level of the vascular ring in order to relieve the stridor. Stridor results from continuous pulsations causing weakening and eventual destruction of the cartilage rings of the trachea.

Case 59.   This neonate was born at 30 weeks' gestation following a difficult delivery.

Questions:

1. Describe the abnormalities on the enhanced computed tomographic scans of the head (C59.1).

2. What is the diagnosis?

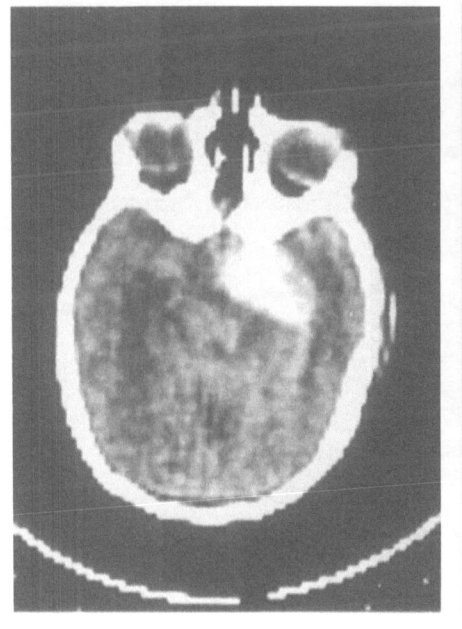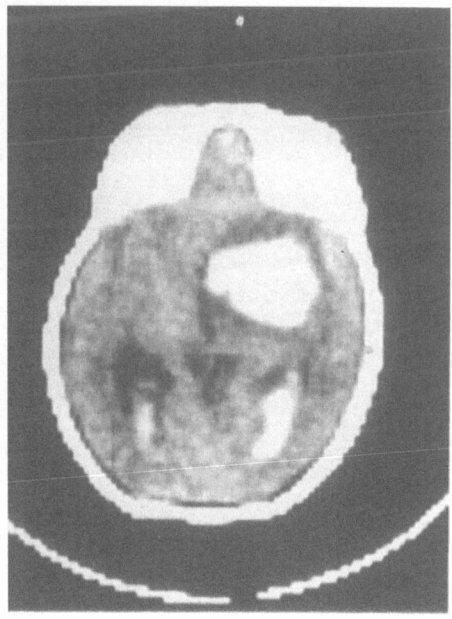

C59.1

Case 59. *Answers:*

1. There are areas of enhancement in the right frontal area and in the dilated lateral ventricles.

2. Intracranial and intraventricular haemorrhage.

Case 59. *Comments:*

C59.2 illustrates the sagittal ultrasound scan on the same neonate, through the right lateral ventricle. The acute area of haemorrhage is echo-dense. Two weeks later the haemorrhage is resolving (C59.3), but there has been significant ventricular dilatation.

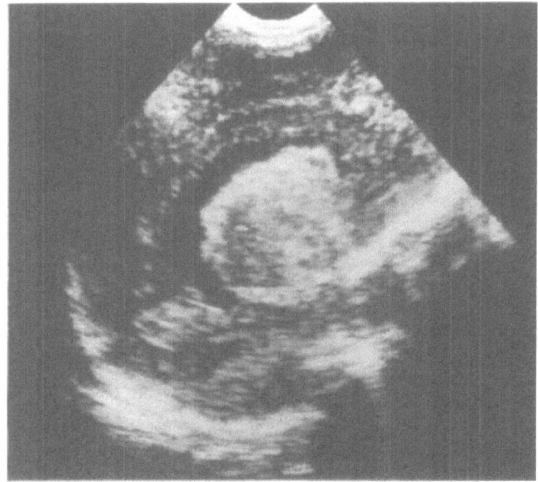

C59.2

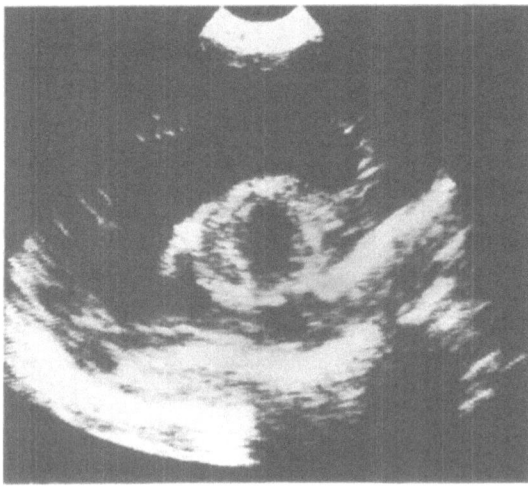

C59.3

Case 60. This is a lateral skull radiograph (C60.1) of a neonate with spinal dysraphism.

Questions:

1. Describe the radiological findings.
2. What is the name given to this appearance?

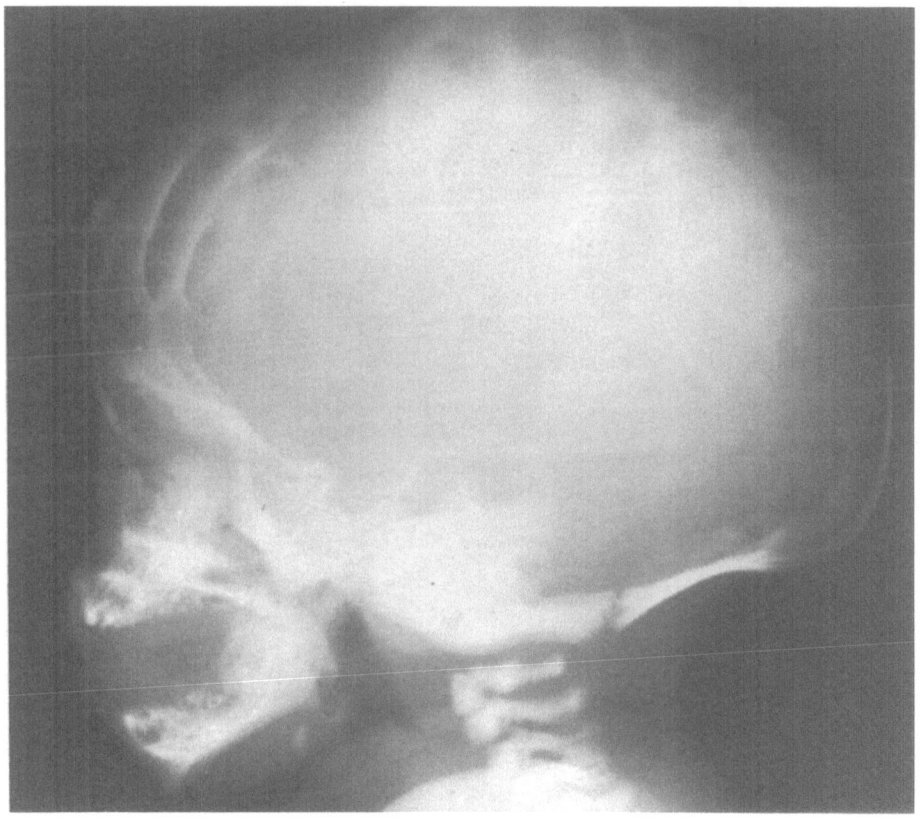

C60.1

Case 60. Answers:

1. There are multiple discrete areas of thinning of the vault bones.
2. A cranio-lacunar skull.

Case 60. Comments:

Cranio-lacunar skull is seen in neonates with spinal dysraphism (usually a lumbar meningomyelocoele) (C60.2). These specific radiological appearances in the skull revert to normal within several months. A cranio-lacunar appearance is not the same as a "copper beaten" appearance, which is seen in the presence of raised intracranial pressure only after the cranial sutures have fused.

Many neonates with meningomyelocoele develop hydrocephalus, the progress of which may be monitored by ultrasound of the head. C60.3 illustrates a coronal scan of symmetrically dilated lateral ventricles (transonic areas). C60.4 is the midline sagittal scan showing dilated lateral and third ventricles.

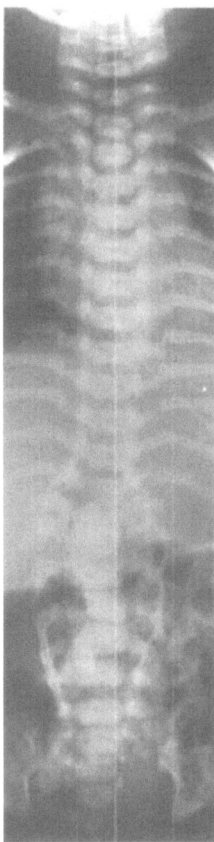
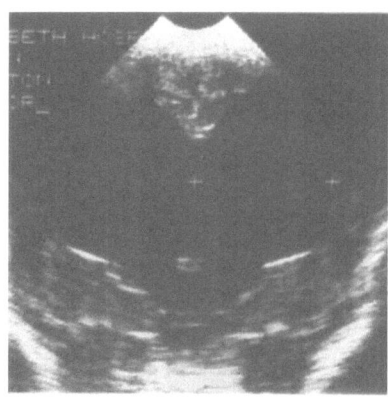
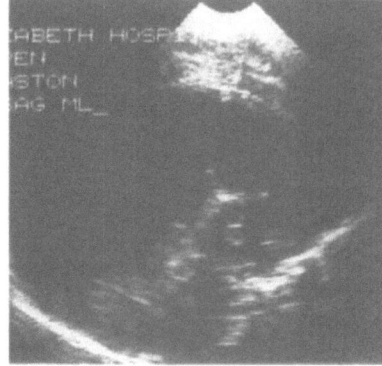

C60.2   C60.4

Case 61.   This 10-year-old girl has short ring and little fingers.

Questions:

1. What is this special examination of the skull (C61.1)?
2. What does it demonstrate?
3. What is the diagnosis?

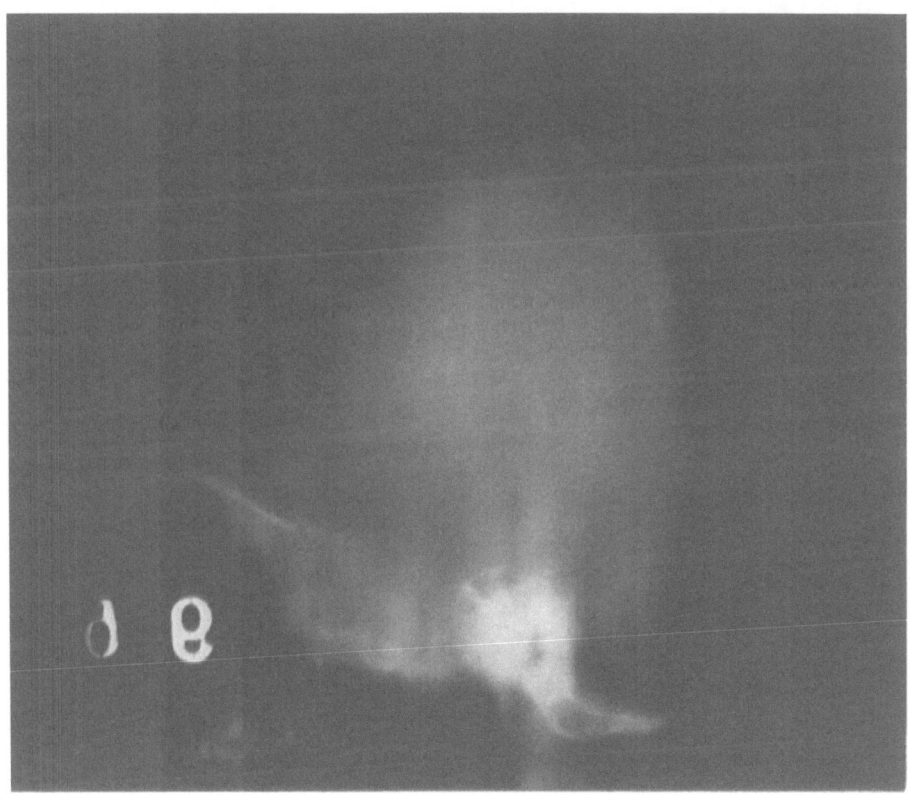

C61.1

Case 61. *Answers:*

1. Lateral tomography.
2. Calcification in the basal ganglia.
3. Pseudohypoparathyroidism.

Case 61. *Comments:*

Basal ganglia calcification is seen in:

a) Pseudohypoparathyroidism—with hypocalcaemia and deficient end-organ responsiveness. Changes of secondary hyperparathyroidism may also be present.

b) Pseudopseudohypoparathyroidism in which blood chemistry is often normal.

c) Mitochondrial cytopathy (myopathy).

Case 62.   This 3-week-old neonate presented with microphthalmia and convulsions.

Questions:

1. Describe the abnormalities on the skull radiograph (C62.1).
2. What is the diagnosis?

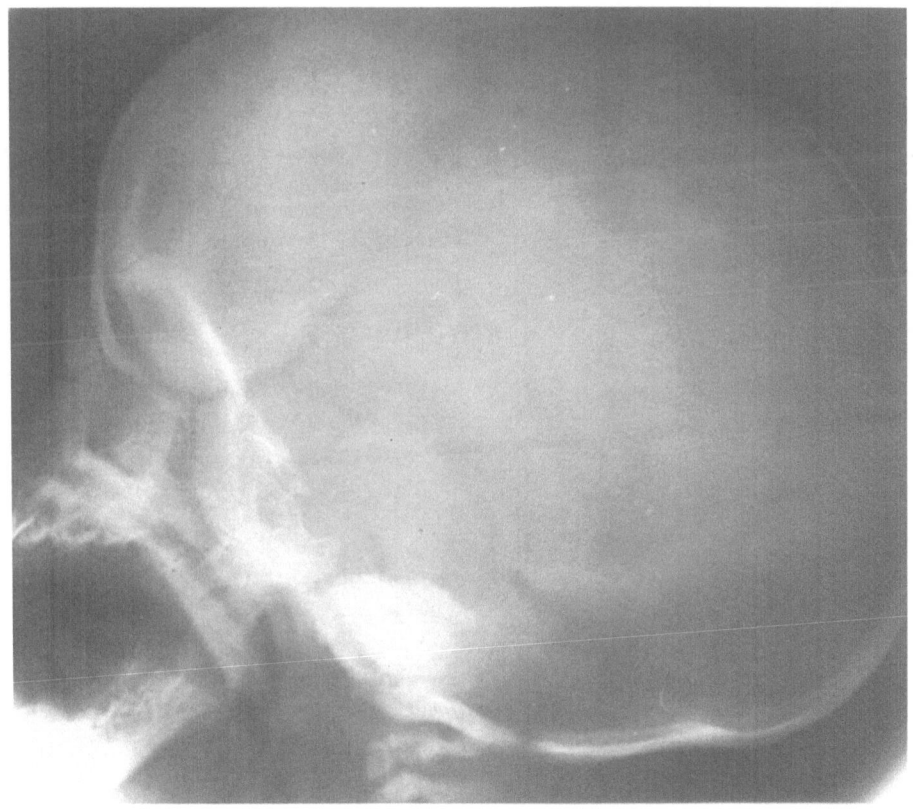

C62.1

Case 62. *Answers:*

1. Scattered curvilinear calcification in clusters.

2. Toxoplasmosis.

Case 62. *Comments:*

Uncooked pork is an important source of infection in man. Other TORCHS infections (rubella, cytomegaloviral infection, herpes and syphilis) do not cause calcifications in the neonate, but they may become apparent later in childhood.

Case 63. This lateral skull radiograph (C63.1) was taken in a child with headaches.

Questions:

1. What could be the cause of the headaches?
2. Why is the skull vault thickened?

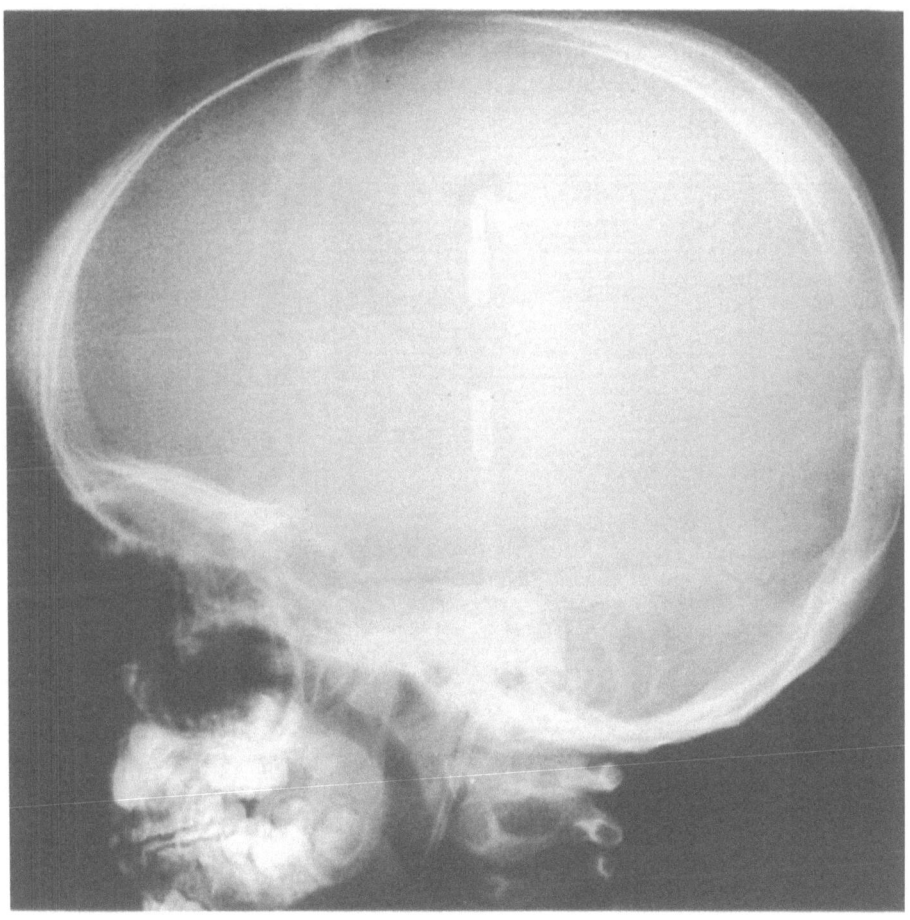

C63.1

Case 63. Answers:

1. Blocked Spitz-Holter valve and raised intracranial pressure.
2. There has been rebound thickening of the vault bones following relief of the hydrocephalus.

Case 64. This neonate was unwell following a stormy delivery. The control film (C64.1) of this IVU examination demonstrated a fine rim of calcification in the right hypochondrium.

Questions:

1. Describe the IVU appearances.
2. What is the differential diagnosis of this radiographic appearance?
3. What is the most likely diagnosis with this clinical presentation?
4. What would you expect to see on a plain abdominal radiograph in 6 years' time?
5. What is the contrast medium of choice for the IVU examination?

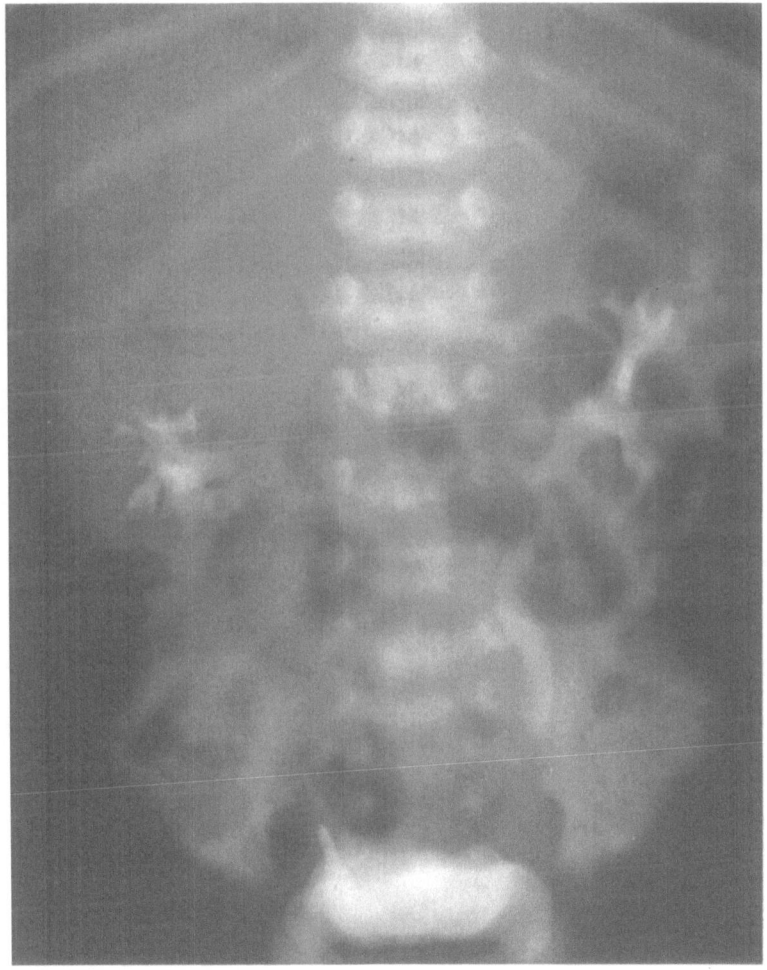

C64.1

Case 64. Answers:

1. Right kidney depressed. Upper pole rotated laterally with a relatively lucent area above the kidney. (Moderately dilated left ureter.)

2. Adrenal haemorrhage; adrenal abscess; obstructed upper pole duplex kidney (but this should not calcify; also the displaced kidney has a normal number of calyces).

3. Adrenal haemorrhage.

4. Adrenal calcification.

5. Non-ionic contrast medium in a neonate to prevent electrolyte imbalance.

Case 65. This is an IVU examination (C65.1) on an infant who presented with failure to thrive and was found to have a palpable left kidney.

Questions:

1. What soft tissue abnormality would have been present on the control film?
2. Why was the left kidney palpable?
3. What is the likely diagnosis?

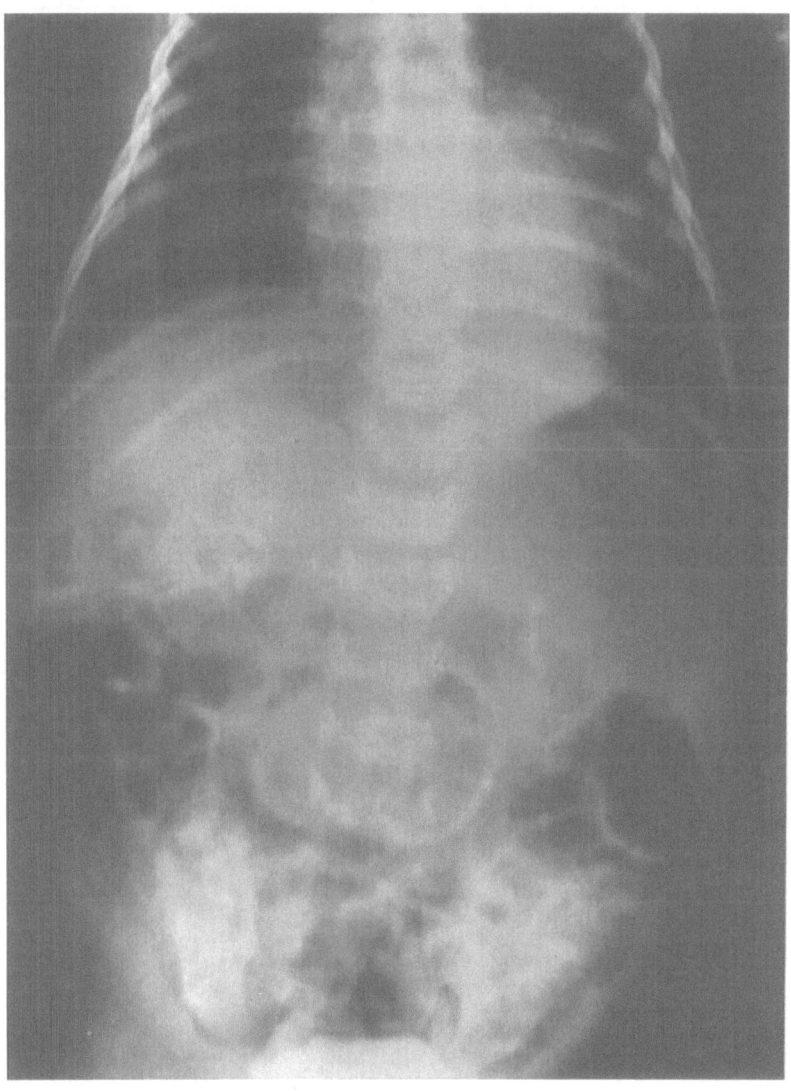

C65.1

Case 65. Answers:

1. A soft tissue mass in the left posterior mediastinum seen separate from and therefore behind the heart shadow.
2. Displaced downwards by the mass extending downwards through the diaphragm.
3. Neurogenic tumour (neuroblastoma).

Case 66. This 5-year-old boy presented with precocious virility and has a bone maturation corresponding to 10 years.

Questions:

1. On this IVU film (C66.1) what is wrong with the right kidney?
2. What abnormalities would be present on the control film?
3. What is the diagnosis?

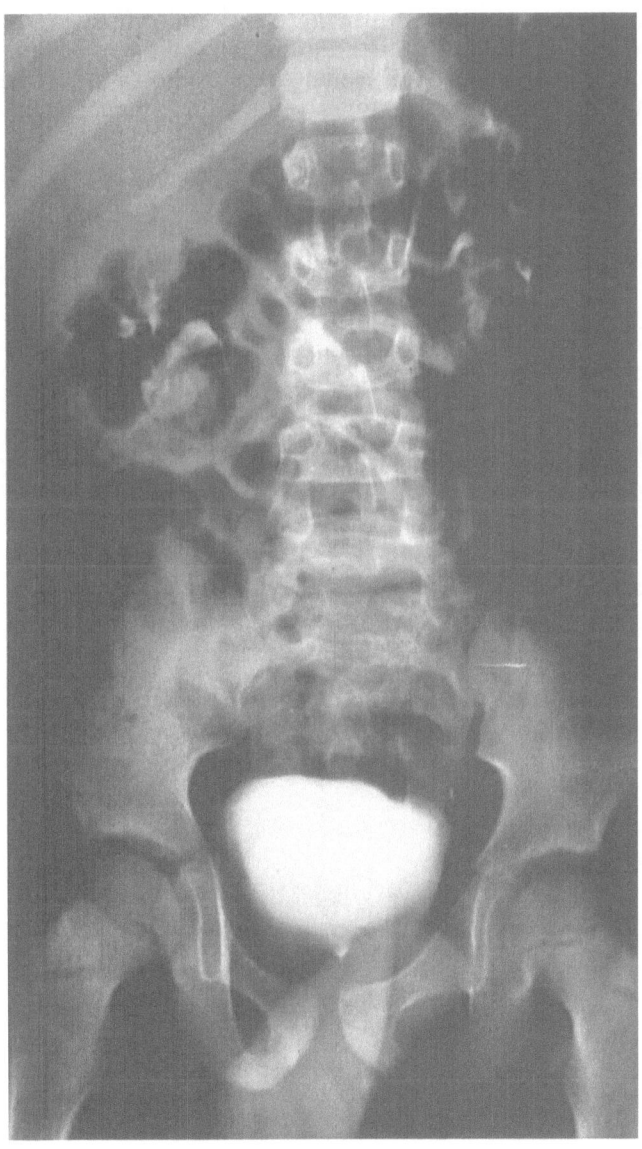

C66.1

Case 66. *Answers:*

1. Displaced downwards with some lateral rotation of the upper pole.
2. Soft tissue mass with speckled "tumour" calcification in the right hypochondrium. Enlargement of the penis.
3. Adrenal cortical carcinoma (not neuroblastoma).

Case 66. *Comments:*

In childhood, adrenal cortical tumours are usually active endocrinologically, resulting in a combination of virilisation and Cushing's syndrome. A large adrenal cortical tumour is more likely to be malignant. Nelson's syndrome (pituitary tumours and hyperpigmentation) may result after adrenal gland/ tumour resection.

Case 67.   This 10-year-old mentally retarded girl has short stature.

Questions:

1. Describe the abnormal features on the pelvic radiograph (C67.1).
2. What is the differential diagnosis of these radiographic appearances?
3. In the presence of short stature what further investigations would you suggest, and why?

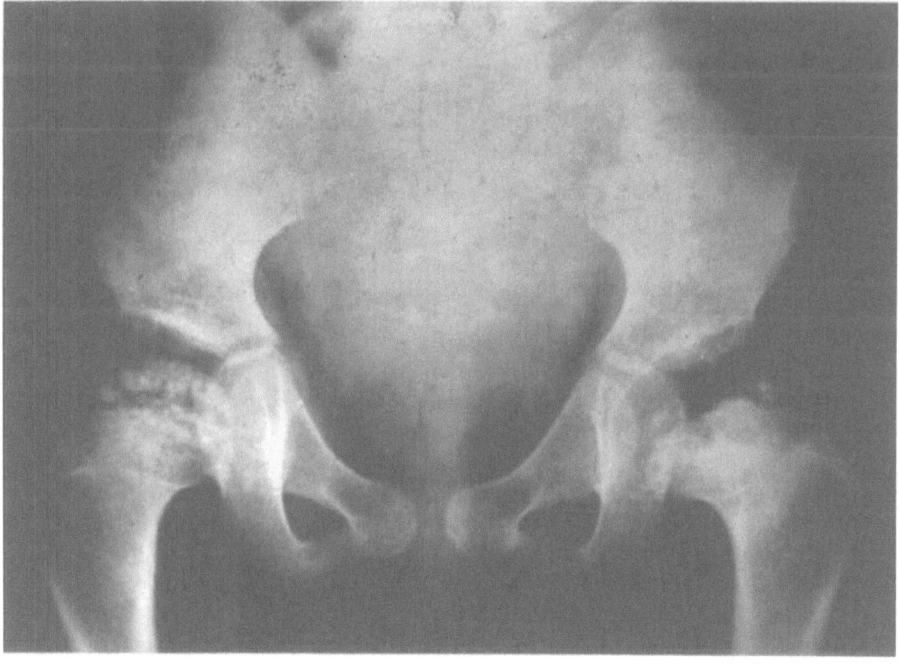

C67.1

Case 67. Answers:

1. There is flattening and fragmentation of both capital femoral epiphyses and the femoral necks are short, broad and in varus.

2. Causes of symmetrical flattening and fragmentation: hypothyroidism; Mayer's isolated dysplasia; skeletal dysplasias (multiple epiphyseal dysplasia, chondrodysplasia punctata, mucopolysaccharidoses and mucolipidoses, hereditary arthro-ophthalmopathy, trichorhino-phalangeal syndrome, spondyloepiphyseal dysplasias). (See list of asymmetrical changes on p. 152)

3. TSH levels and radionuclide scanning for thyroid assessment. Skeletal survey to differentiate dysplasias.

Case 67. Comments:

This girl has hypothyroidism and shows characteristic changes in the spine (C67.2) with a kyphosis and inferior "hooks" on L2 and L3 with a "bone-in-a-bone" appearance. The lateral view of the knee shows delayed maturation and irregular, stippled epiphyses (C67.3). Hypercalcaemia may be a complication.

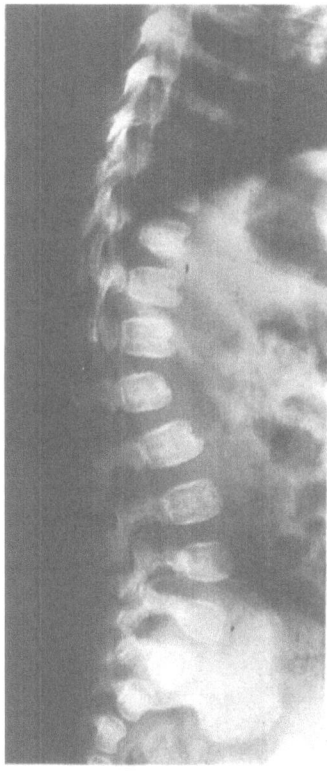

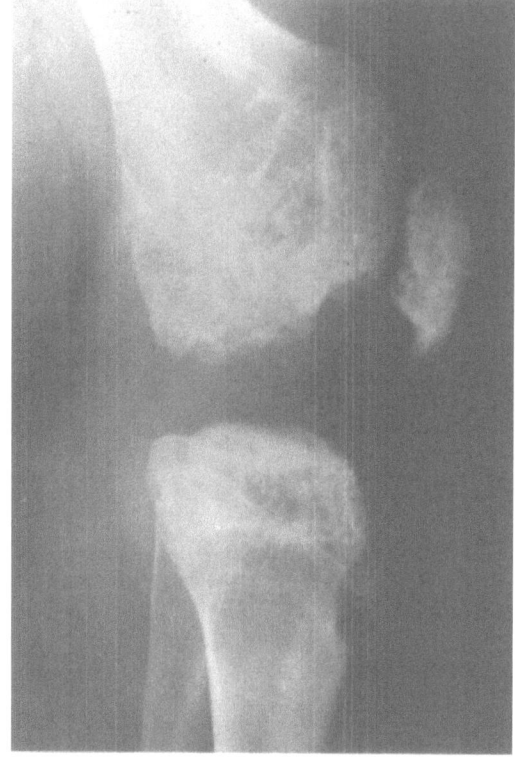

C67.2   C67.3

Case 68. This 5-year-old boy presented with a lump in his neck.

Questions:

1. Describe the abnormality on this lateral neck radiograph (C68.1).
2. What other investigations would be appropriate, and why?
3. What is the differential diagnosis?

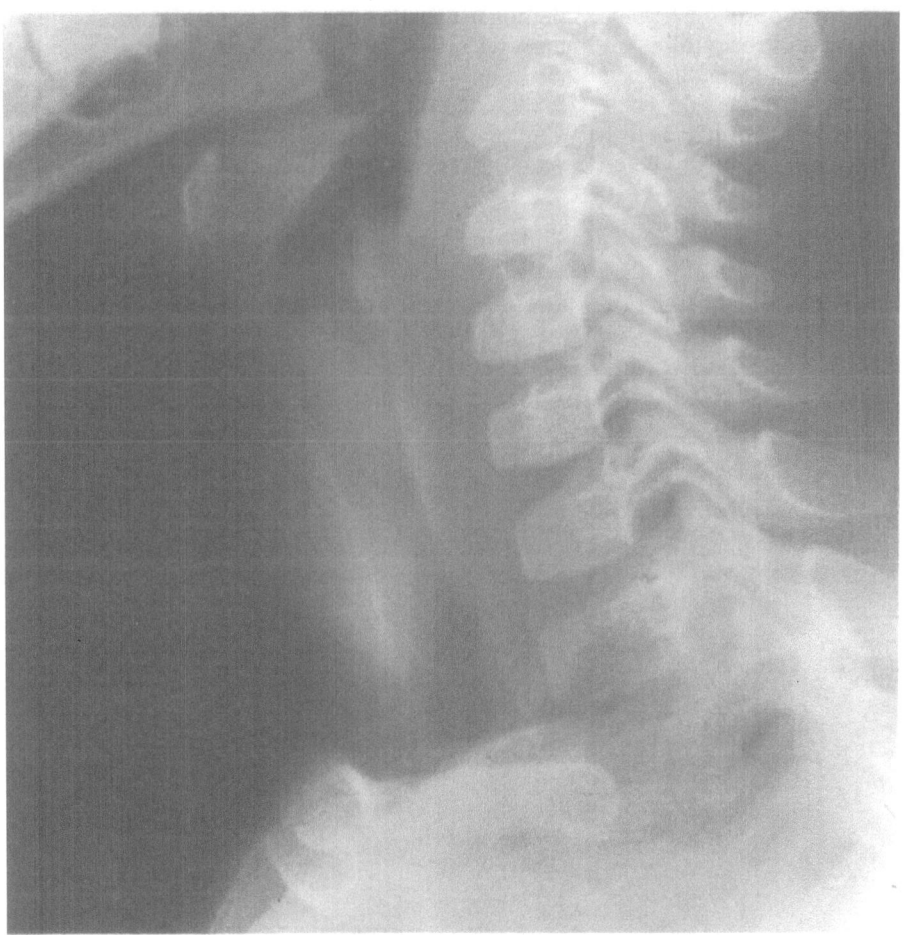

C68.1

Case 68. Answers:

1. There is a clearly defined soft tissue mass in front of the trachea.

2. a) Ultrasound to determine whether the mass (probably thyroid) is solid or cystic, solitary or multiple nodules.
   b) Radionuclide study to determine the presence or absence of active thyroid tissue.
   c) Biopsy under ultrasound control.
   d) Chest radiograph (miliary shadowing is a feature of metastatic thyroid carcinoma).

3. Thyroid carcinoma (final diagnosis); thyroglossal cyst; goitre; auto-immune thyroiditis.

Case 68. Comments:

The ultrasound scan (C68.2) demonstrates that the mass is solid, solitary, lies to the right of the midline and measures about 3 cm in diameter. (Multiple nodules are rarely malignant.)

The radionuclide scan (C68.3) demonstrates the midline marker in the suprasternal notch, active thyroid tissue to the left of the midline (side without the mass) and also higher, normal excretion from the salivary glands.

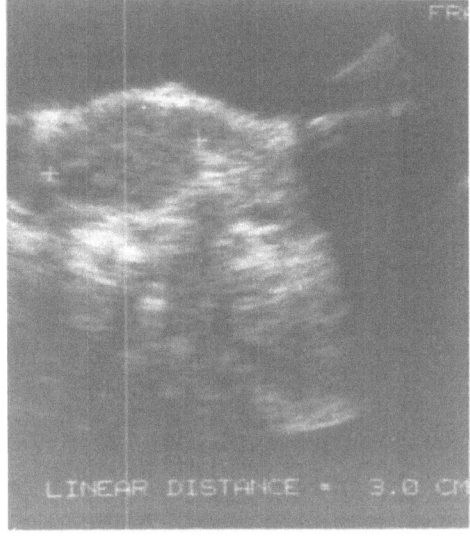

C68.2

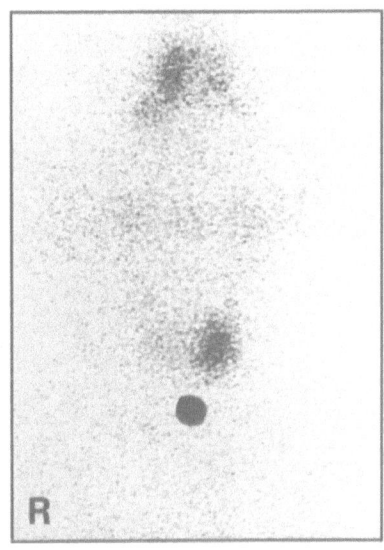

C68.3

Case 69.   This 10-year-old girl presented with pain and a soft tissue swelling over the left chest wall.

Questions:

1. Describe the soft tissue changes (C69.1).
2. Describe the bony changes.
3. What is the differential diagnosis?

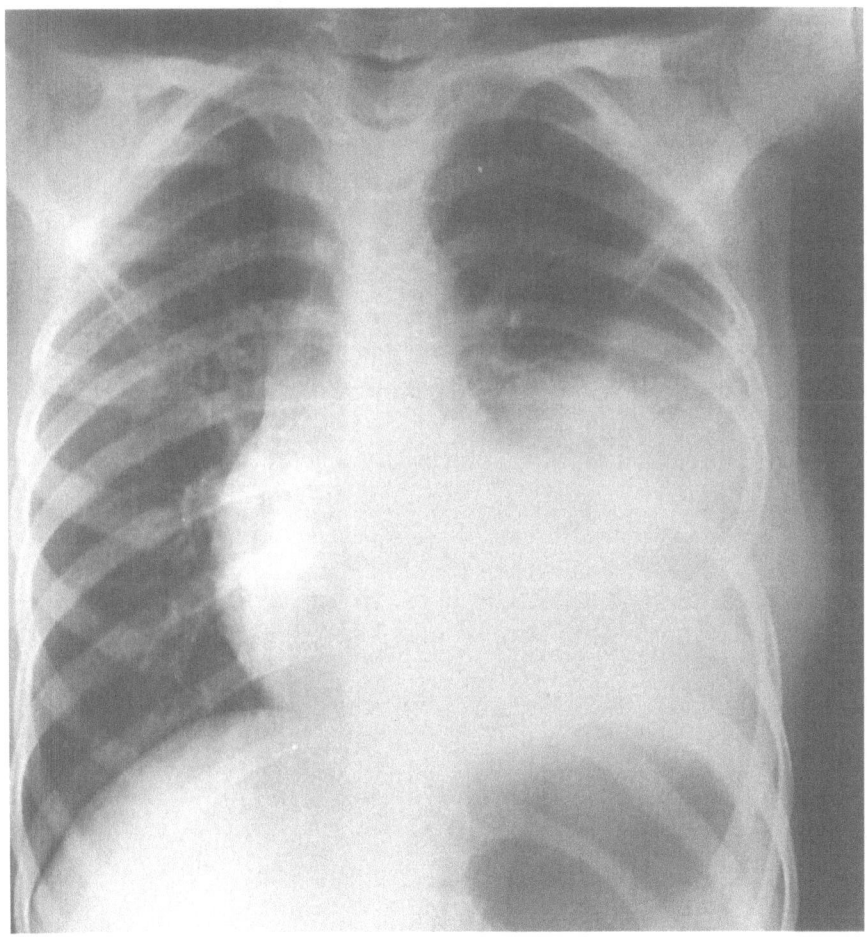

C69.1

Case 69.   Answers:

1. Homogeneous soft tissue shadowing over the left mid and lower zones is probably intra- and extra-pleural. Also soft tissue swelling over the inferior angle of the left scapula is present. The soft tissue planes are preserved, but displaced.

2. Destruction of the middle third of the left sixth rib.

3. Ewing's sarcoma (final biopsy diagnosis); aneurysmal bone cyst; tuberculosis (but adjacent ribs appear normal).

Case 69.   Comments:

The preservation but displacement of soft tissue planes indicates tumour mass (benign or malignant) rather than infection.

Case 70. These are AP (C70.1) and lateral (C70.2) radiographs of the right knee of a 10-year-old boy. He had pain here for 3 weeks and had started to limp.

Questions:

1. Describe the bony abnormalities.

2. Describe the soft tissue abnormalities.

3. What is the diagnosis?

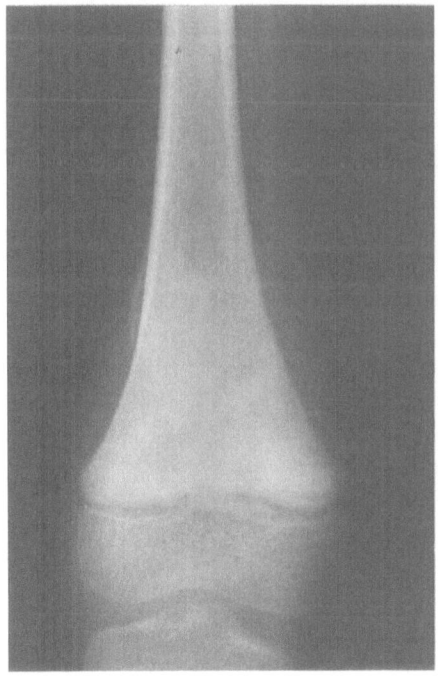

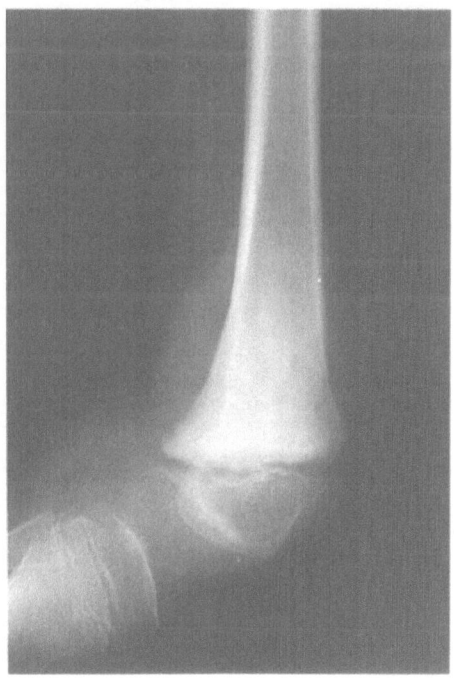

C70.1   C70.2

Case 70.   Answers:

1. Sclerosis in the region of the metaphysis, extending into the diaphysis, with an ill-defined margin and a periosteal reaction.

2. The soft tissue planes are preserved but are displaced by a soft tissue mass.

3. Osteosarcoma.

Case 70.   Comments:

The soft tissue planes would be lost in the presence of an infective process. Ewing's sarcoma more commonly affects the diaphysis.

Case 71. This 6-year-old boy presented with otitis media, a painful swelling of the left forearm and a painful shoulder.

Questions:

1. Describe the appearances of the skull vault (C71.1).

2. What is the diagnosis?

3. What is the descriptive term sometimes used for this radiographic appearance?

4. What radiographic appearances would indicate the healing phase?

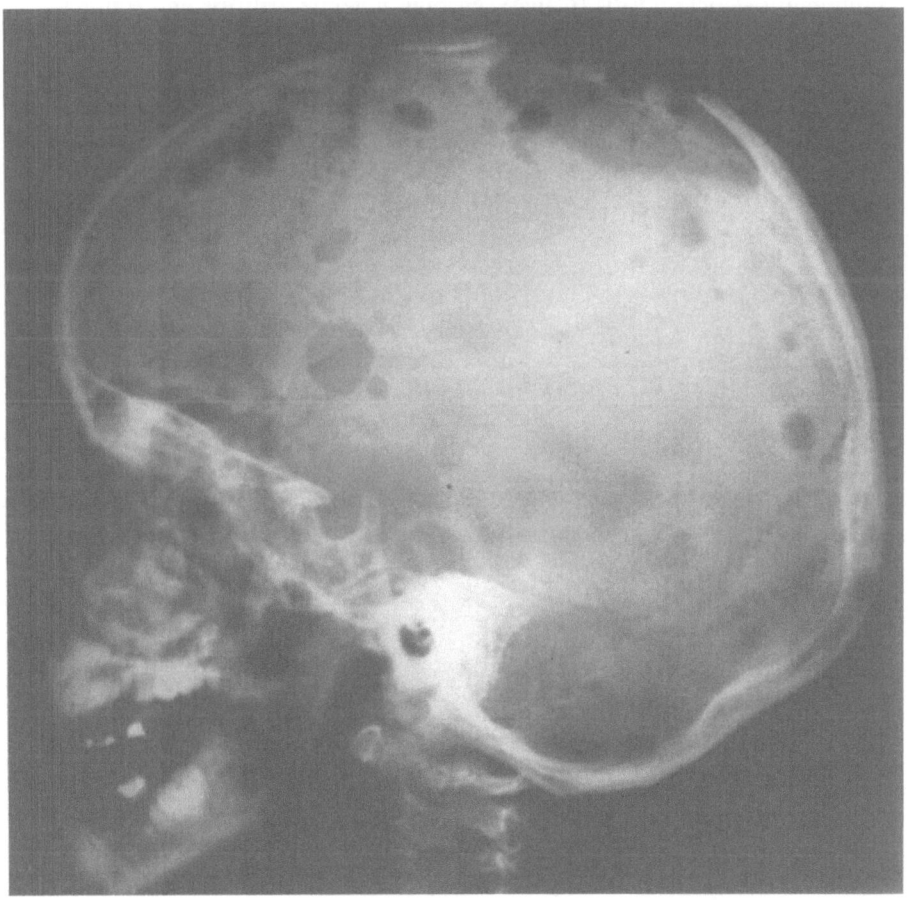

C71.1

Case 71. Answers:

1. There are multiple "punched-out" lytic areas with destruction of the inner and outer tables.
2. Eosinophilic granuloma.
3. A "geographical" skull.
4. A sclerotic margin to the lytic areas.

Case 71. Comments:

Eosinophilic granuloma in the long bones may be diaphyseal and may be associated with expansion, erosion, periosteal new bone formation and overlying soft tissue swelling. Occasionally metaphyses and epiphyses are affected. In the spine a single collapsed vertebra (vertebra plana) may be present (C71.2). Other causes of this appearance include leukaemia, neuroblastoma, lymphoma, osteochondritis (Calvé), chronic juvenile arthritis and trauma.

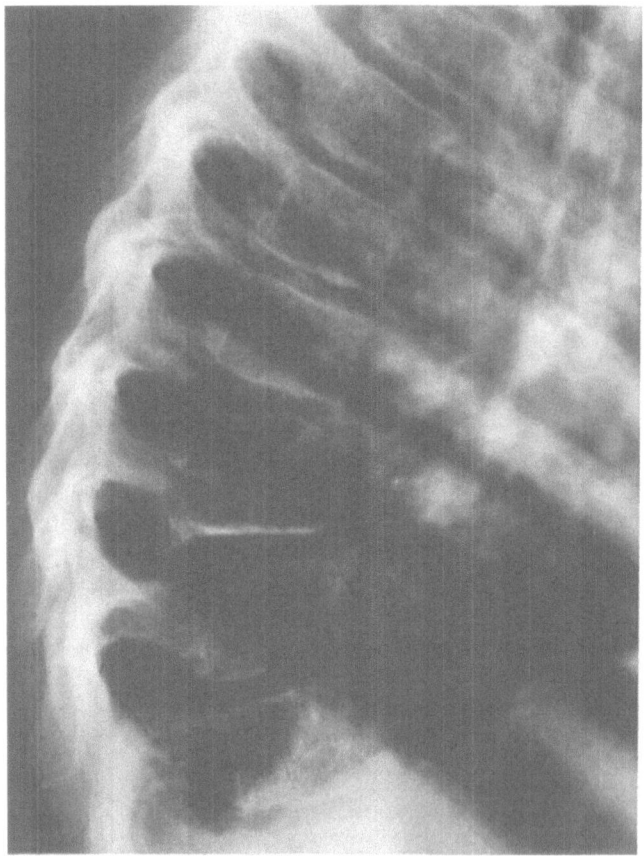

C71.2

Case 72.   This 4-year-old boy presented with a history of lethargy and bone pain lasting several months. He had sustained pathological fractures of the left tibia and right femur. An abdominal mass was palpable.

Questions:

1. Describe the radiological changes in the skull vault (C72.1).

2. What is the diagnosis?

3. What is the differential diagnosis for this skull appearance?

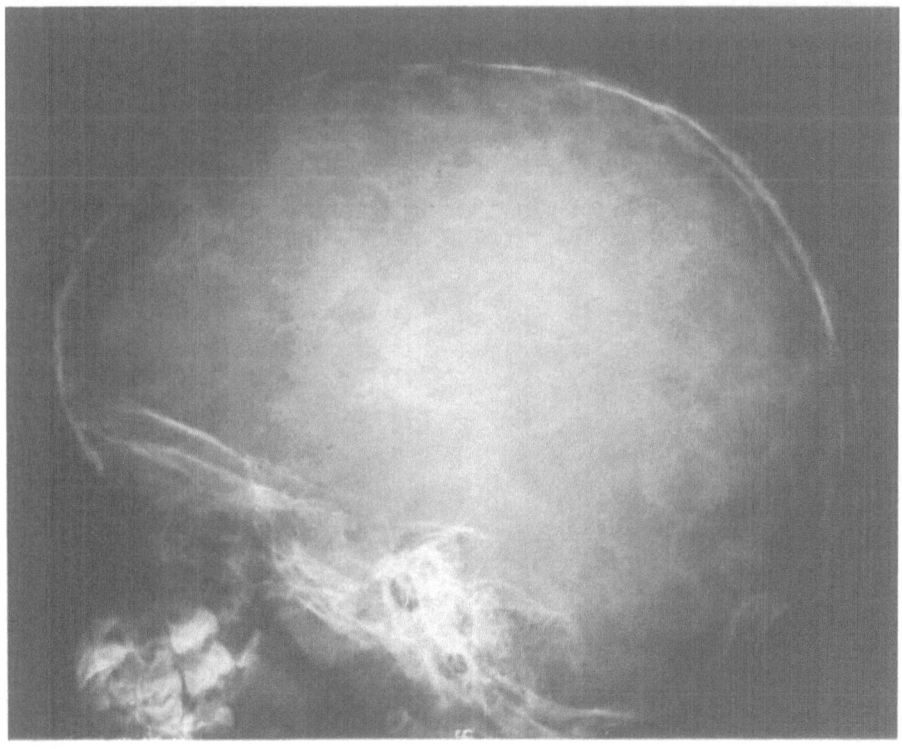

C72.1

Case 72.   Answers:

1. There is irregular patchy lysis involving the whole vault. Marked interdigitations of the coronal suture are present.

2. Neuroblastoma with metastatic spread to bone.

3. Leukaemia—a skull radiograph of a 4-year-old boy with leukaemia is illustrated (C72.2).

Case 72.   Comments:

In both neuroblastoma and leukaemia there may be metastatic involvement of the sutures. Also raised intracranial pressure may occur.

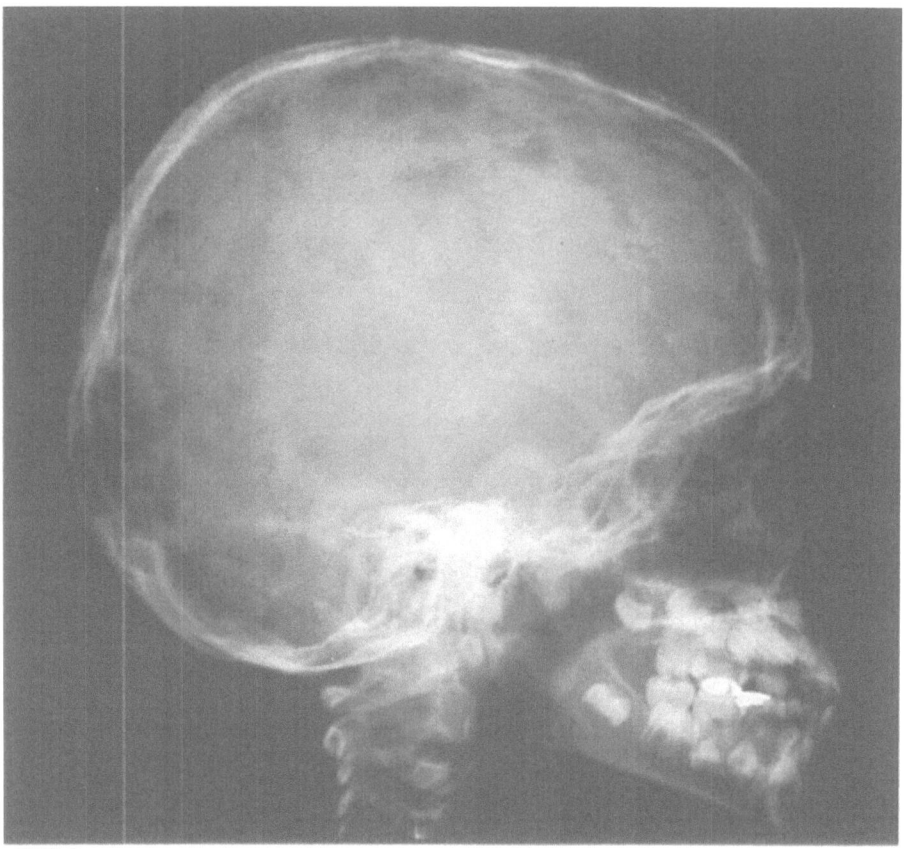

C72.2

Case 73. This 10-year-old boy presented with pain in his legs and a pathological fracture through his tibial metaphysis.

Questions:

1. Describe the bony abnormalities on the pelvic radiograph (C73.1).
2. What is the differential diagnosis?

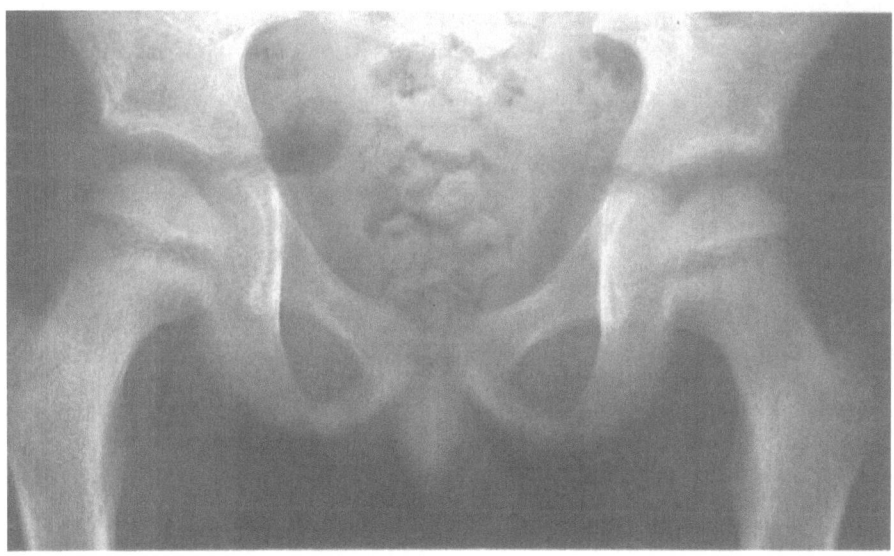

C73.1

Case 73.   Answers:

1. There is osteoporosis with coarsening of the trabecular pattern. Apparent widening of the epiphyseal plates caused by radiolucent bands at the metaphyses is present. There are periosteal reactions around the pelvic ring and along the right femoral neck.

2. Rickets, metastatic leukaemia (final diagnosis), or neuroblastoma.

Case 73.   Comments:

More clearly defined metaphyseal radiolucent bands may be present in the healing phase of rickets. C73.2 illustrates the wrist of a child who had been receiving anti-tuberculous therapy and had developed rickets.

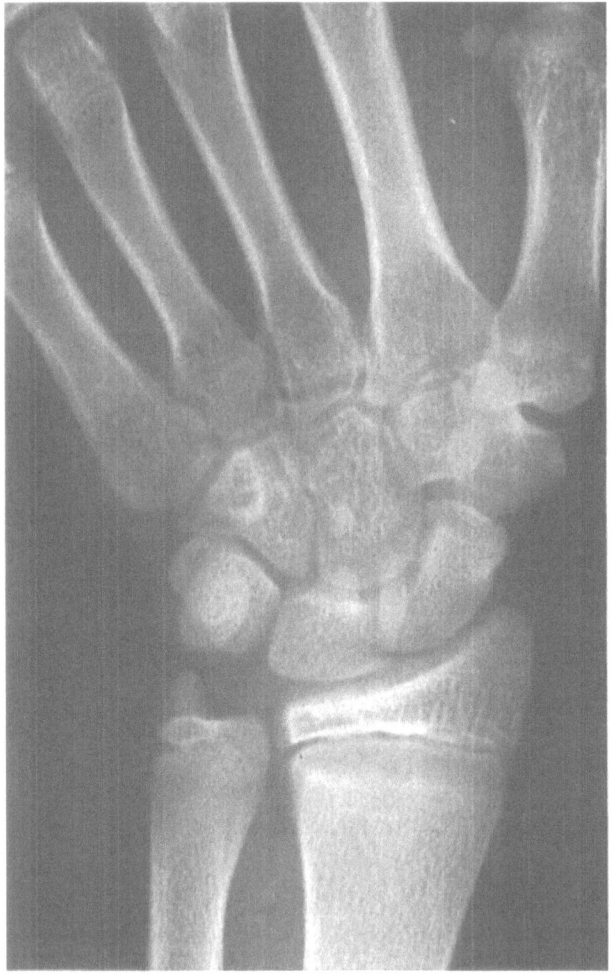

C73.2

Case 74. This 5-year-old boy presented with pain and swelling of the right lower leg of 1 month's duration. An AP (C74.1) radiograph of the ankle was obtained.

Questions:

1. Which part of the tibia is involved?
2. Describe the bony changes.
3. What is the differential diagnosis?

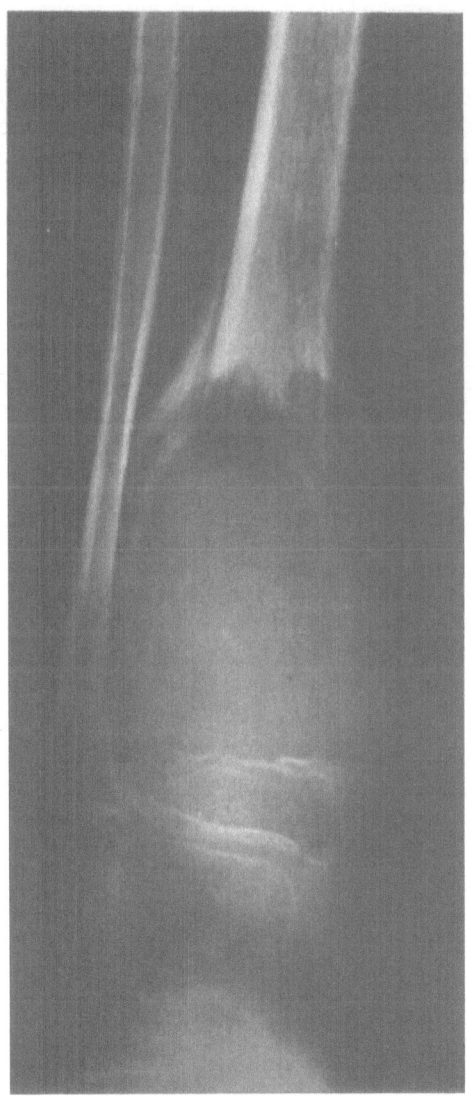

C74.1

Case 74. *Answers:*

1. The distal tibial metaphysis.
2. Bone expansion with lysis; cortical destruction; periosteal new bone formation; clearly defined zone of transition.
3. Osteomyelitis; tumour—benign; tumour—malignant.

Case 74. *Comments:*

The degree of bone expansion and cortical destruction without any associated sclerosis and the preservation (but displacement) of soft tissue planes are against a diagnosis of osteomyelitis. The zone of transition is too clearly defined for this to be a malignant bone tumour. Also the periosteal new bone formation, when a response to adjacent cortical destruction, is not necessarily a feature of malignancy. This was a benign aneurysmal bone cyst. Very few benign bone tumours give this degree of expansion and cortical destruction. Note the marked osteoporosis distal to the aneurysmal bone cyst.

Case 75. **This 9-year-old boy presented with pain in his hip of several months' duration.**

Questions:

1. Describe the abnormality on the left hip radiograph (C75.1).
2. What is the differential diagnosis?
3. What further investigations may be of value?

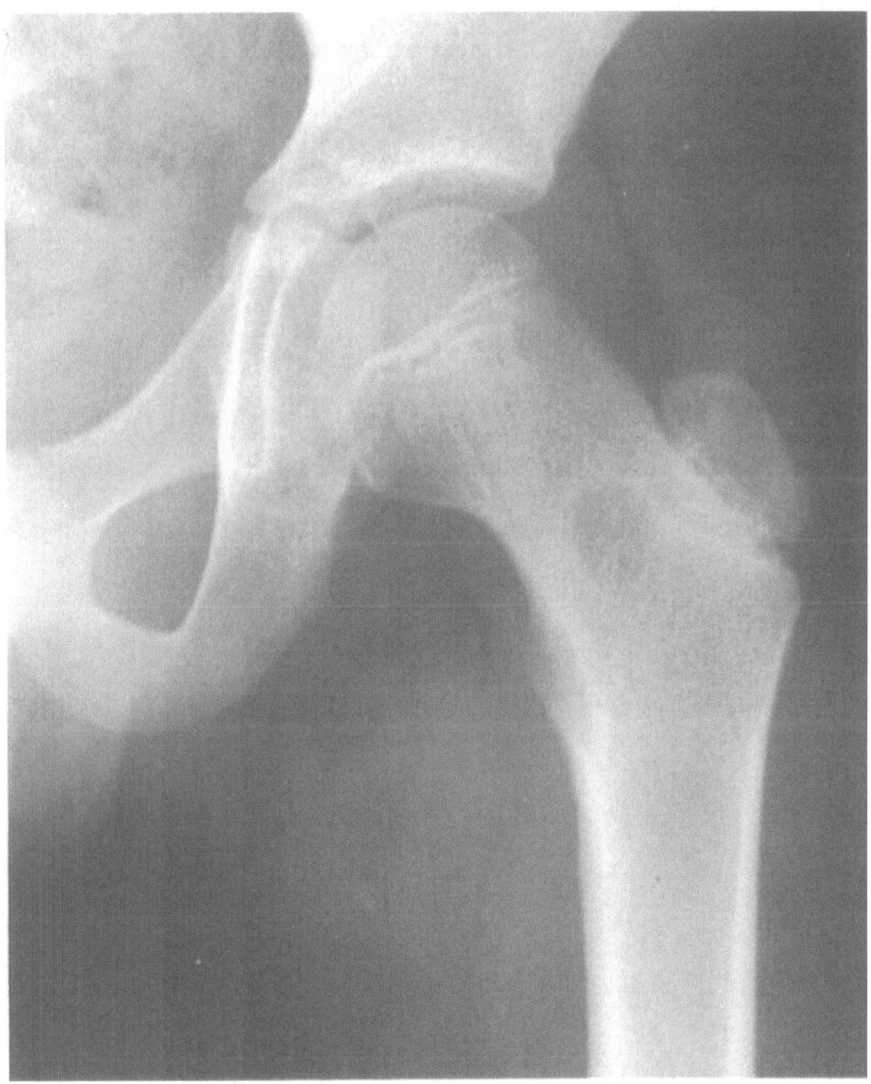

C75.1

Case 75. *Answers:*

1. There is a clearly defined, rounded radiolucent area 1 cm in diameter in the femoral neck. It has a sclerotic margin.
2. Brodie's abscess; osteoid osteoma (final diagnosis); simple bone cyst; osteoblastoma; fibrous cortical defect; eosinophilic granuloma.
3. View of other hip; tomography; radionuclide Tc^{99m} bone scan; biopsy.

Case 75. *Comments:*

The radionuclide bone scan (C75.2) demonstrates localised increased uptake of isotope at the site of the nidus of the osteoid osteoma.

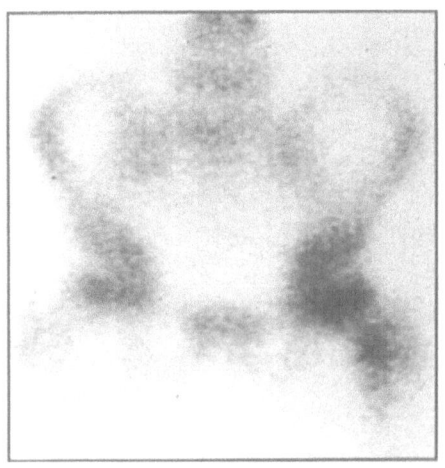 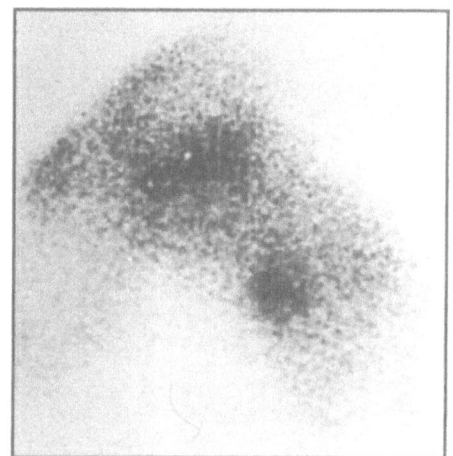

C75.2

Case 76. **This 6-year-old boy presented with pain in the right hip and a limp.**

Questions:

1. a) Describe the changes of the right hip joint (C76.1).
   b) Describe the changes of the right capital femoral epiphysis.
   c) Describe the changes of the right upper femoral metaphysis.

2. What is the most likely diagnosis?

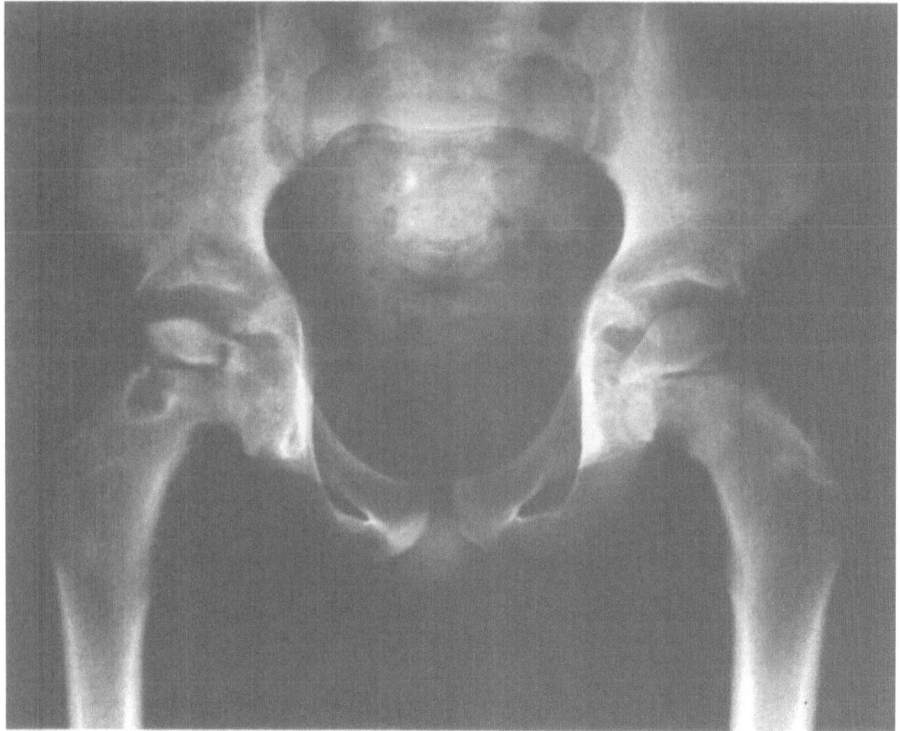

C76.1

Case 76. *Answers:*

1. a) The joint space is widened.
   b) Flattened, fragmented and sclerotic.
   c) Widened with radiolucent defects.

2. Perthes' disease.

Case 76. *Comments:*

Differential diagnosis of unilateral avascular necrosis of a capital femoral epiphysis includes: Perthes' disease; sickle-cell disease; steroid therapy; post-radiation necrosis; trauma (manipulation for congenitally dislocated hips); Gaucher's disease; leukaemia; haemophilia; and homocystinuria.

In these conditions, although the changes may be bilateral they are usually asymmetrical.

Case 77. This negro child of 10 years had multiple episodes of painful joints, initially affecting her hips. She now presents with a painful left shoulder.

Questions:

1. Describe the changes in the proximal humeral epiphysis (C77.1).
2. What is the likely underlying etiology?
3. List the skeletal abnormalities which may be found in this condition.

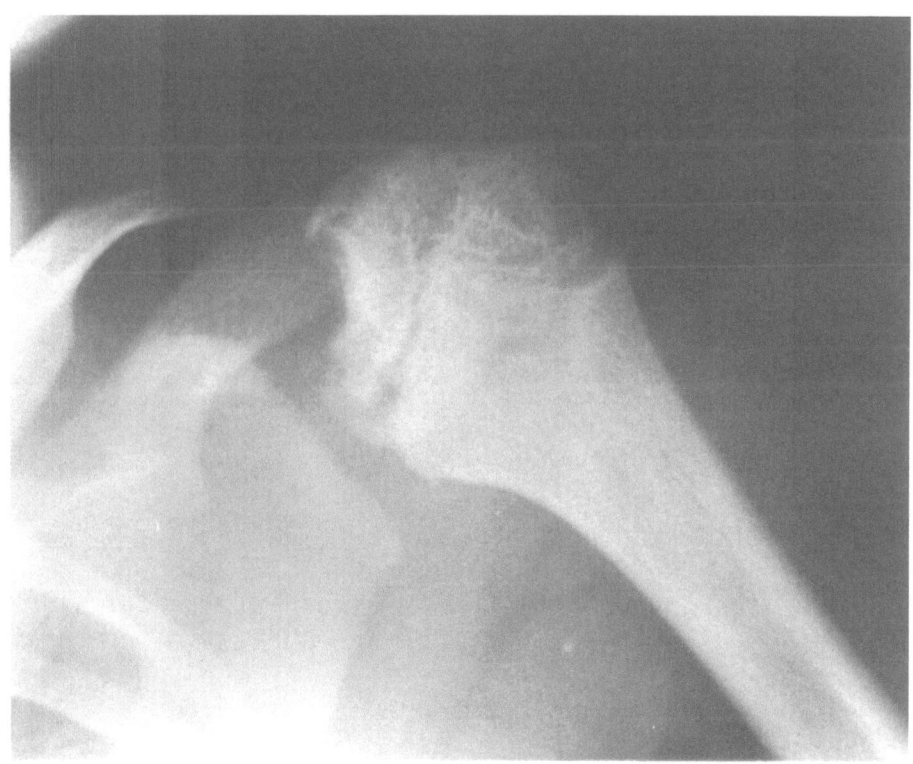

C77.1

Case 77.   Answers:

1. Flattening, fragmentation and sclerosis of the epiphysis with articular irregularity (the "snow-cap" appearance).

2. Ischaemic necrosis due to sickle-cell disease.

3. Dactylitis in infancy (C77.2); ischaemic necrosis of epiphyses—also affecting the vertebral end-plates, causing a "step" deformity (C77.3); bone infarcts; salmonella osteomyelitis (characteristically diaphyseal) (C77.4).

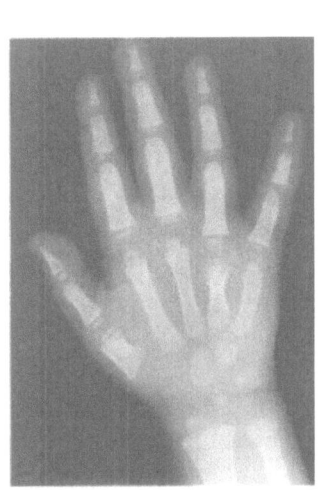

C77.2

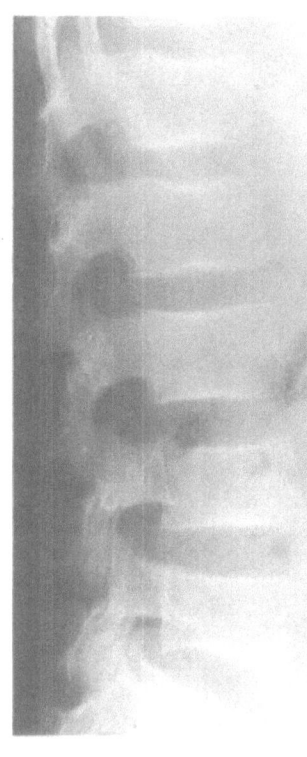

C77.3

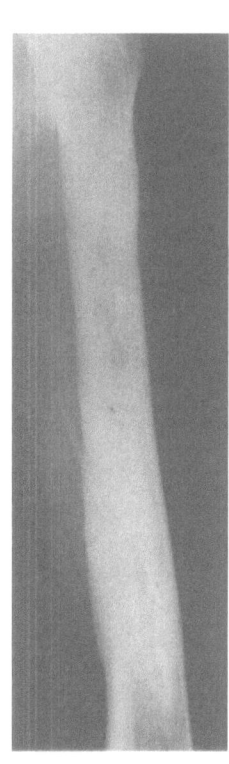

C77.4

Case 78. This 5-year-old boy presented with lethargy and was found to be anaemic.

Questions:

1. Describe the appearances of the skull vault (C78.1).
2. Describe the appearances of the facial bones.
3. What is the diagnosis?

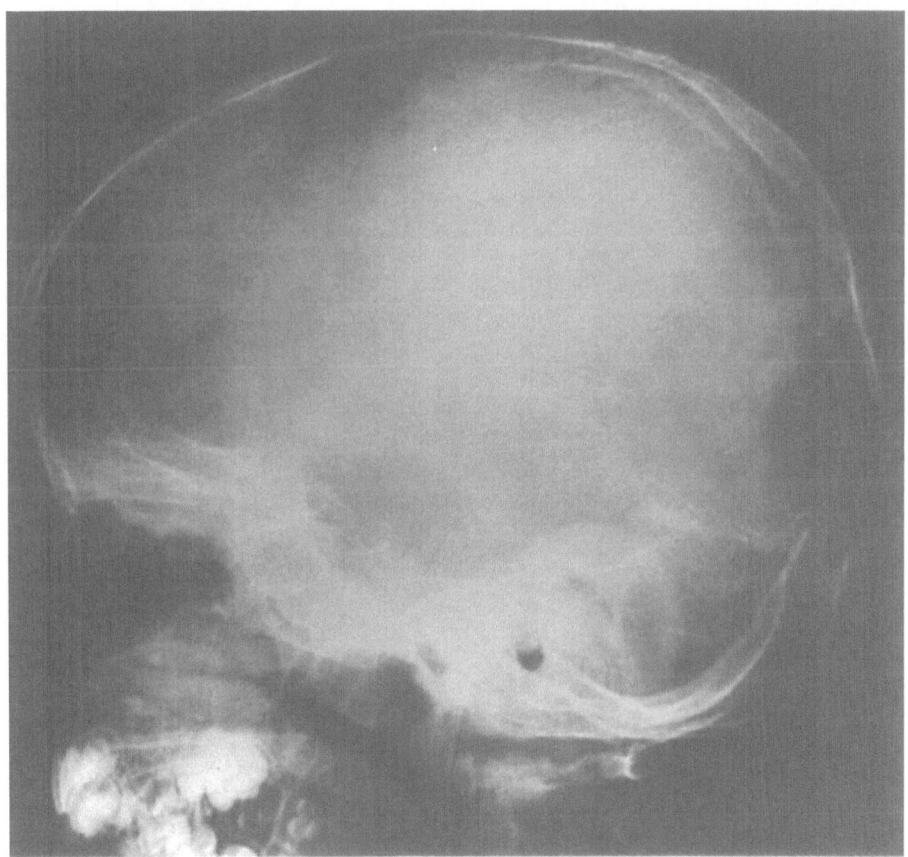

C78.1

Case 78. Answers:

1. Widening of the diploic space with thinning of the inner and outer tables.
2. There is no aeration of the maxillary antra, sphenoid or frontal sinuses, due to extramedullary haemopoiesis.
3. Thalassaemia major.

Case 78. Comments:

C78.2 illustrates the "hair-on-end" appearance which is also seen in this condition.

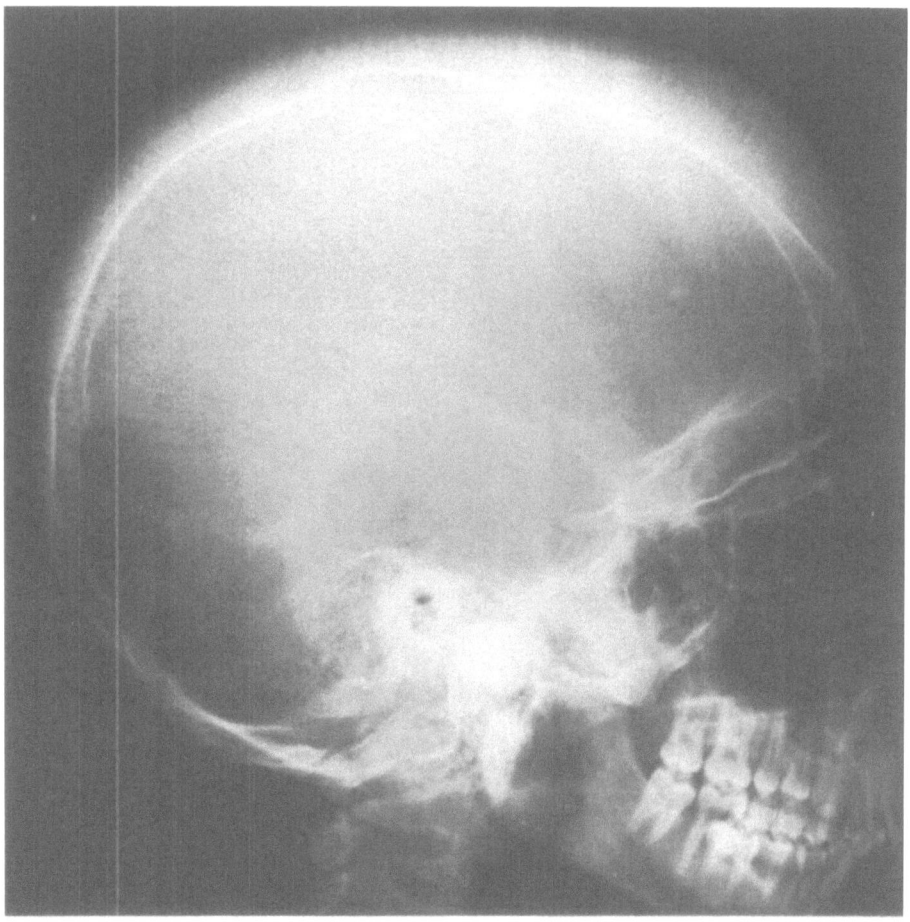

C78.2

Case 79. This 10-year-old girl presented with neck pain and stiffness. She had had recurrent episodes of joint pain over the previous 2 years.

Questions:

1. Describe the abnormalities on the flexion (C79.1) and extension (C79.2) views of the cervical spine.
2. What is the likely diagnosis?
3. What are the radiological features of this disorder?
4. Which areas of the skeleton are affected maximally?

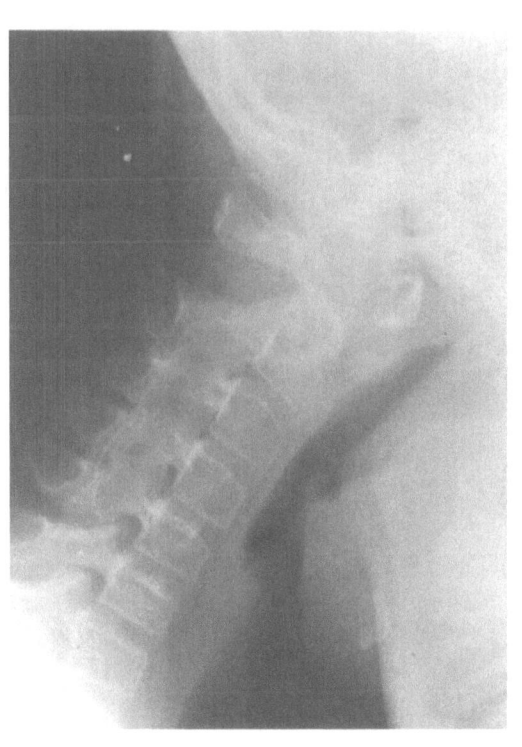

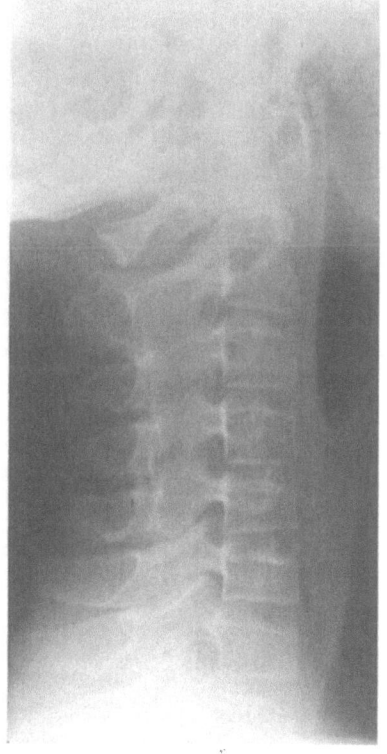

C79.1   C79.2

Case 79. Answers:

1. Flexion and extension are limited due to fusion of the laminae from C2 to C5. There is generalised osteoporosis. At the C5 to C6 apophyseal joint there is some sclerosis with joint space narrowing; probable early spondylosis related to excessive movement at this level.

2. Chronic juvenile arthritis (rheumatoid arthritis/Still's disease).

3. Osteoporosis, especially in the periarticular regions; joint space narrowing and erosions of articular surfaces; joint capsular swelling; later bone destruction, ankylosis and flexion contractures; advanced, but later retarded, bone maturation.

4. Single large joints; small joints of hands and feet; apophyseal joints in the cervical spine; temporo-mandibular joints.

Case 79. Comments:

C79.3 illustrates end-stage changes; flexion contractures; soft tissue wasting; erosions; carpal fusion.

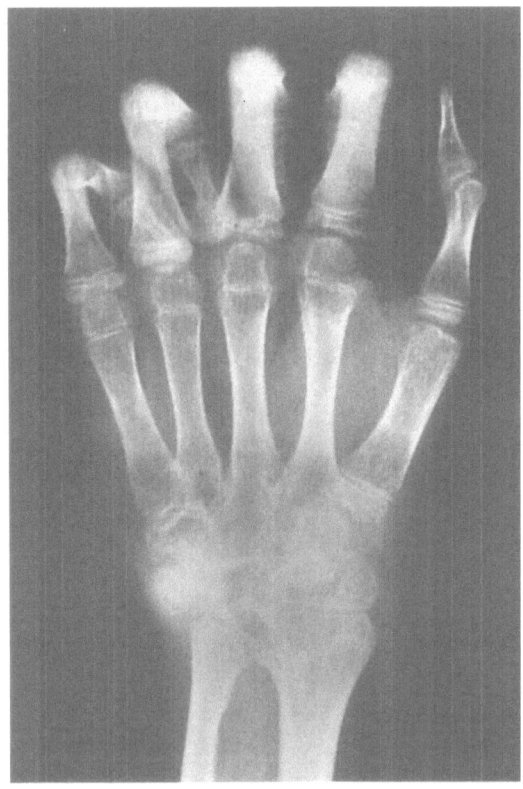

C79.3

Case 80. This 9-year-old boy has had multiple episodes of joint pain. In the past these had been related to minor trauma.

Questions:

1. Describe the abnormal findings at the hips (C80.1).
2. Describe the abnormal findings at the knees (C80.2).
3. What is the differential diagnosis?

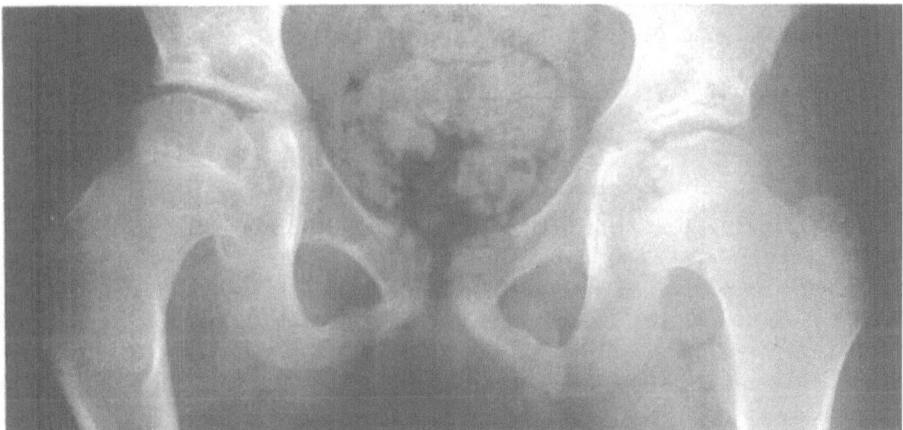

C80.1

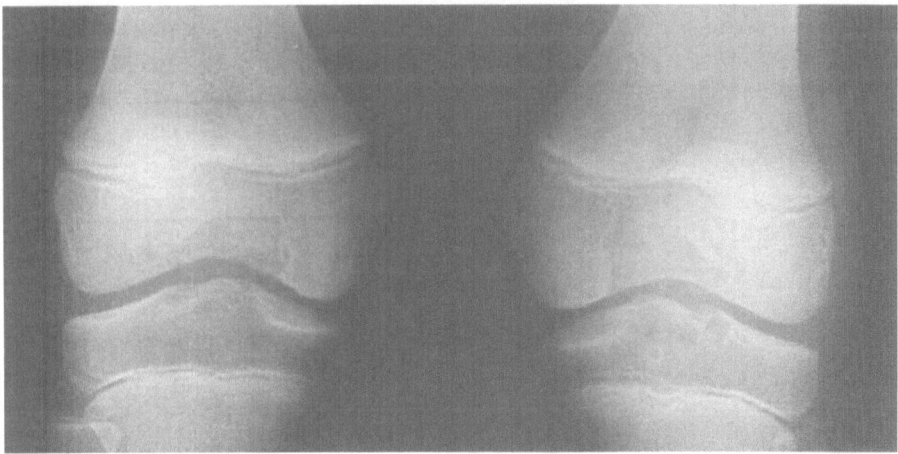

C80.2

Case 80.   Answers:

1. Joint space narrowing; osteoporosis; articular erosions on the capital femoral epiphyses.
2. Articular erosions, with deepening and widening of the intercondylar notches. Capsular swelling, more marked around the left knee.
3. Bleeding disorder (haemophilia) (final diagnosis); chronic juvenile arthritis.

Case 80.   Comments:

C80.3 illustrates an unusual example of an haemophiliac pseudo-tumour caused by subperiosteal bleeding.

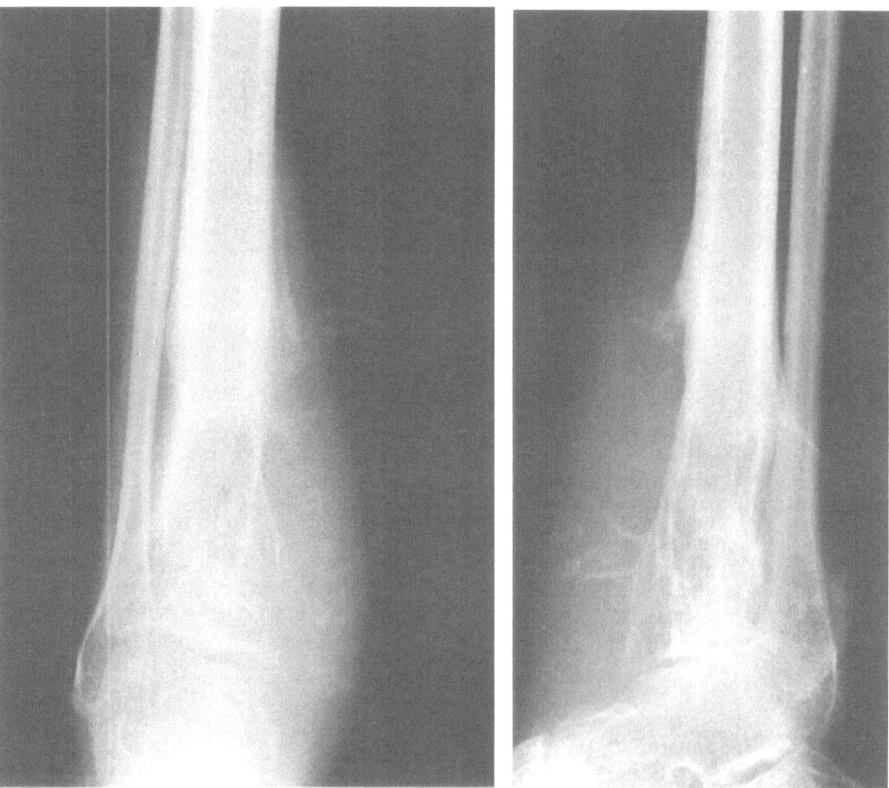

C80.3

Case 81. This 8-year-old girl has chronic renal failure secondary to reflux and severe bilateral pyelonephritis.

Questions:

1. Describe the changes at the epiphyseal plates (C81.1)
2. What are they due to?
3. Are the bones of normal density?
4. This girl does not show evidence of one important feature of renal osteodystrophy. What is this?

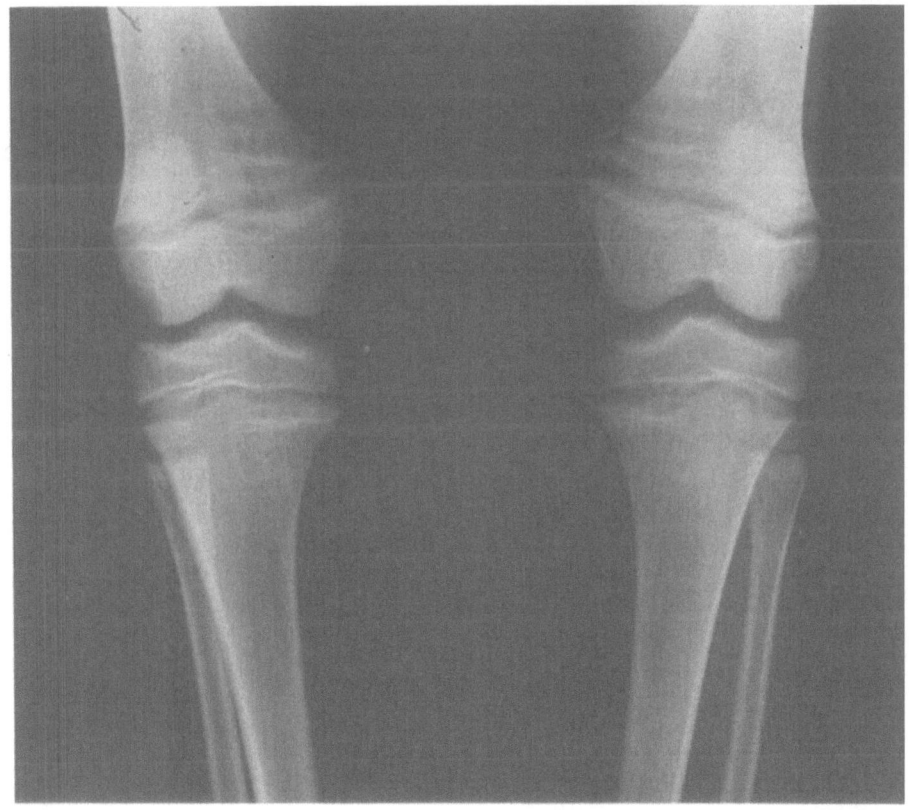

C81.1

Case 81. Answers:

1. There is apparent widening and irregularity.
2. Rickets.
3. No—there are alternating bands of increased and decreased bone density.
4. Secondary hyperparathyroidism (C81.2) with subperiosteal bone resorption which is best seen along the phalangeal diaphyses.

Case 81. Comments:

Other changes of rickets are present—splaying, cupping and fraying of the metaphyses, mild bowing deformities and genu varum. The sclerotic bands in the metaphyses represent evidence of intermittent healing of the rachitic process.

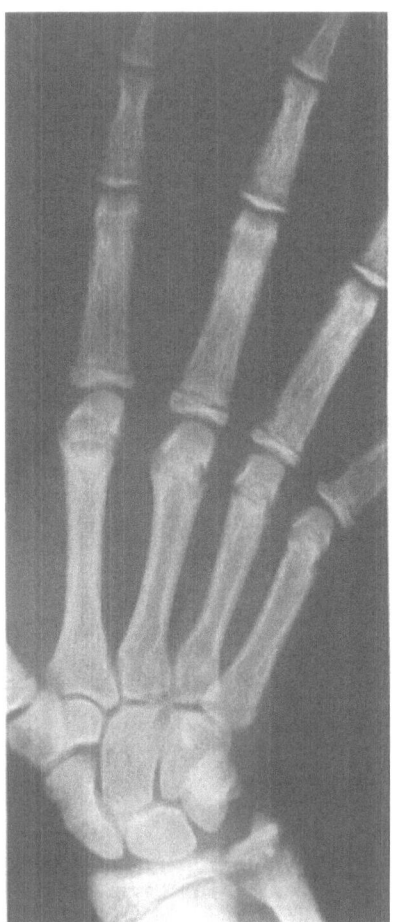

C81.2

Case 82. This 18-month-old negro boy presented with a severe bow-leg deformity.

Questions:

1. Describe the changes at the proximal tibial metaphyses (C82.1).

2. What is the name given to this condition?

3. Are there changes of rickets?

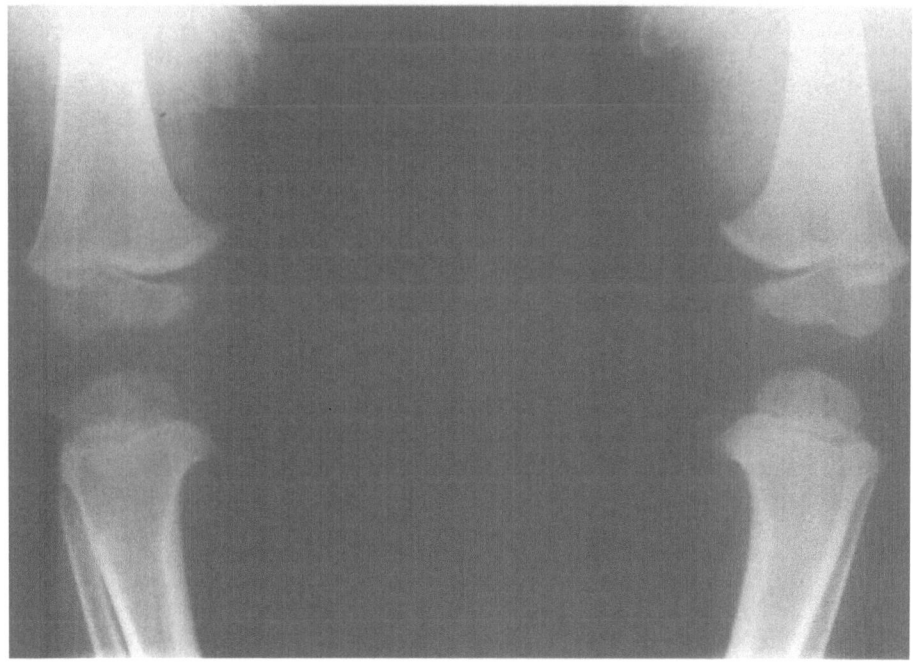

C82.1

Case 82. Answers:

1. Flaring and irregular ossification of the beaked medial metaphyseal angles.
2. Blount's disease.
3. No.

Case 82. Comments:

Other causes of bilateral bow-leg deformities include: rickets; Schmid metaphyseal chondrodysplasia; other skeletal dysplasias with tibio-fibular disproportion, e.g. achondroplasia; intrauterine bowing; idiopathic.

Case 83. This 3-year-old Indian boy presented with a 3-week history of lethargy followed by back pain.

Questions:

1. Describe the abnormalities on the plain (C83.1) and tomographic (C83.2) views of the lateral lumbar spine.
2. What further imaging investigations may be of value?
3. What is the likely diagnosis?

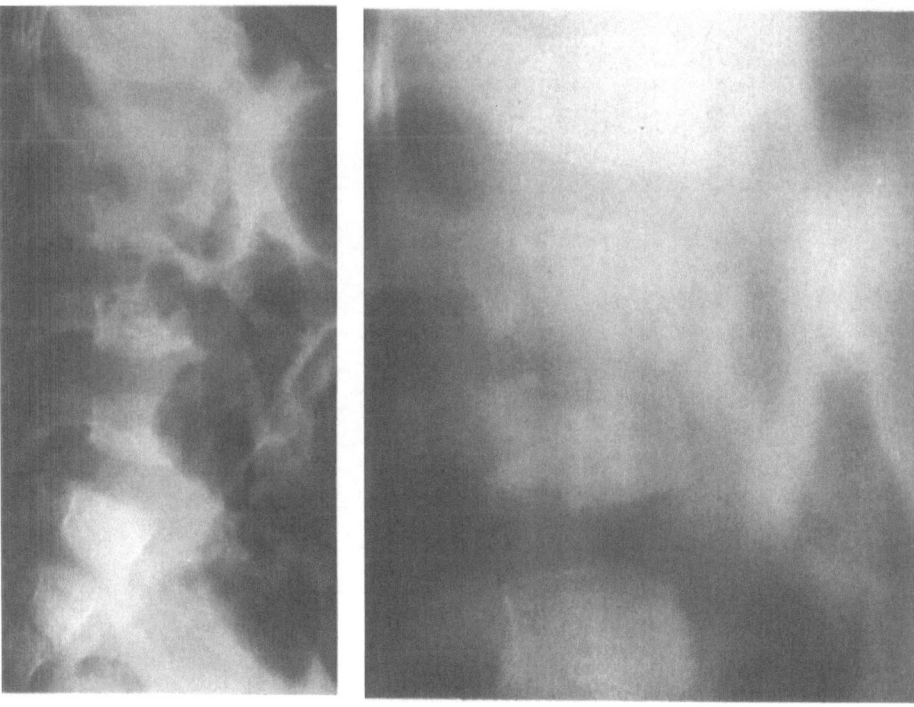

C83.1   C83.2

165

Case 83. Answers:

1. Both views demonstrate loss of height of the L2–L3 disc space with some irregularity of the adjacent vertebral end-plates.

2. a) Radionuclide bone scan. C83.3 demonstrates increased uptake of isotope at L2 and L3 with loss of the disc space here.
   b) Computed tomography (C83.4) demonstrates patchy destruction of the intervertebral disc with a little soft tissue encroachment into the spinal canal. The contrast enhanced aorta has been displaced forwards and there is loss of definition of the paravertebral psoas outlines. C83.5 demonstrates patchy destruction of the adjacent vertebral body.

3. Infection, probably tuberculous in view of involvement of adjacent vertebral bodies.

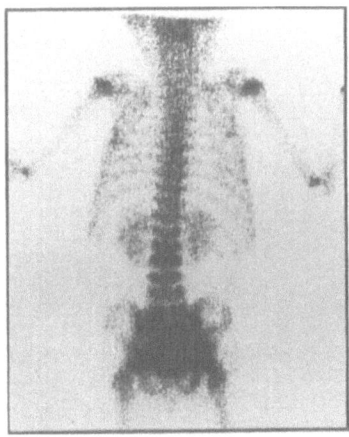

C83.3

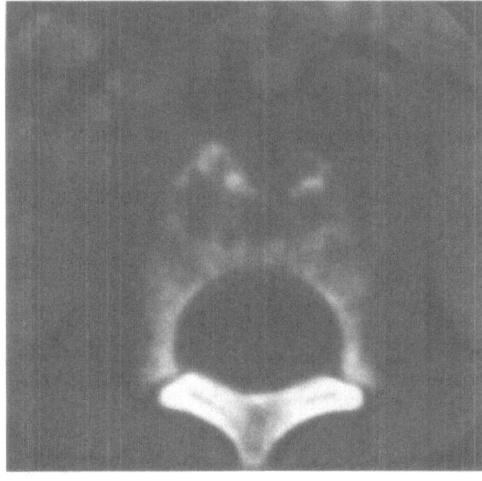

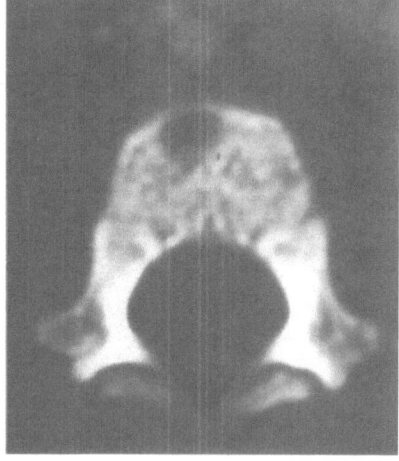

C83.4   C83.5

Case 84. **This boy, now aged 10 years, has chronic lung disease and vomiting. He presented initially as an infant with failure to thrive and recurrent chest infections and at 1 year of age with a painful swollen right hand.**

Questions:

1. Describe the abnormalities on the chest radiograph (C84.1).
2. Describe the abnormalities in the right hand (C84.2).
3. What is the differential diagnosis of the hand appearance?
4. What condition is this boy suffering from and what is the likely cause of his vomiting?

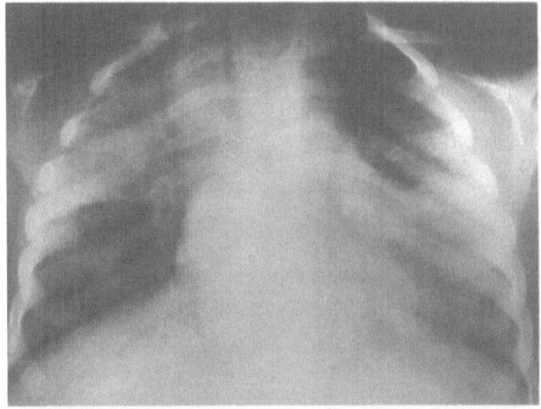

C84.1

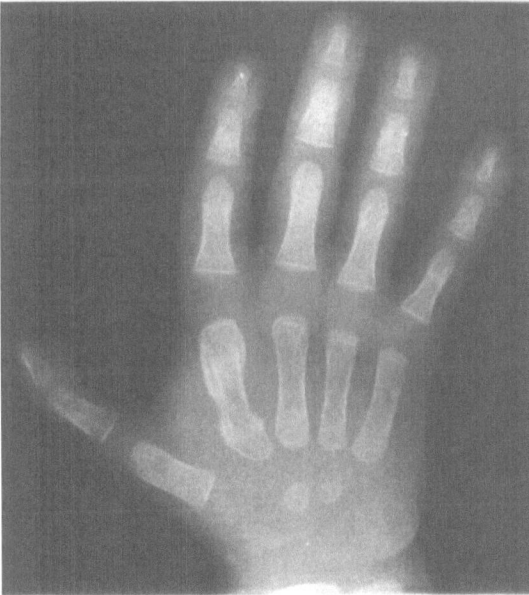

C84.2

Case 84. Answers:

1. There is consolidation in the right upper and left lower zones. The mediastinum is widened.

2. There is periosteal cloaking of the second metacarpal.

3. a) Osteomyelitis
   b) Sickle dactylitis (infection/infarction)
   c) Tuberculous dactylitis

4. Chronic granulomatous disease (The "lazy leucocyte syndrome"). A retroperitoneal fibrosis gives rise to a rigid constriction of the gastric antrum and duodenal loop with hold-up here. Also a mediastinitis causes the oesophagus to be dilated and fixed with an open gastro-oesophageal junction. Changes similar to Crohn's disease may be present in the terminal ileum.

Case 84. Comments:

C84.3 demonstrates old osteomyelitis of the right tenth rib and left iliac crest. Calcification is evidence of an old hepatic abscess.

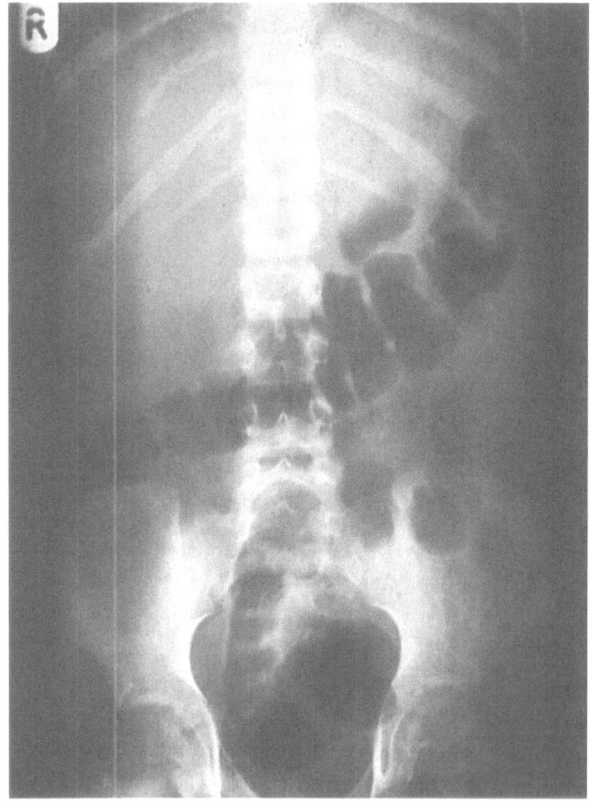

C84.3

Case 85. This 8-year-old boy presented with a painful left hip and a limp.

Questions:

1. Describe the left femoral abnormalities as seen on the pelvic radiograph (C85.1) and left hip arthrogram (C85.2).

2. How may computed tomography of the hips be of value?

3. List the causes of an irritable hip.

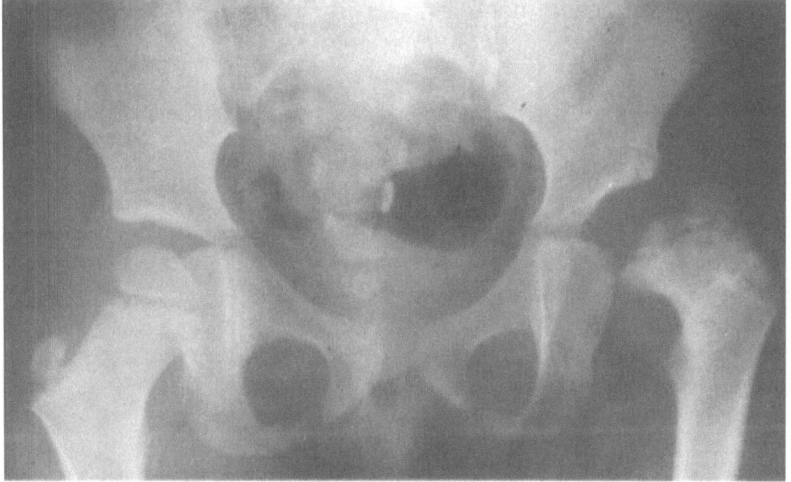

C85.1

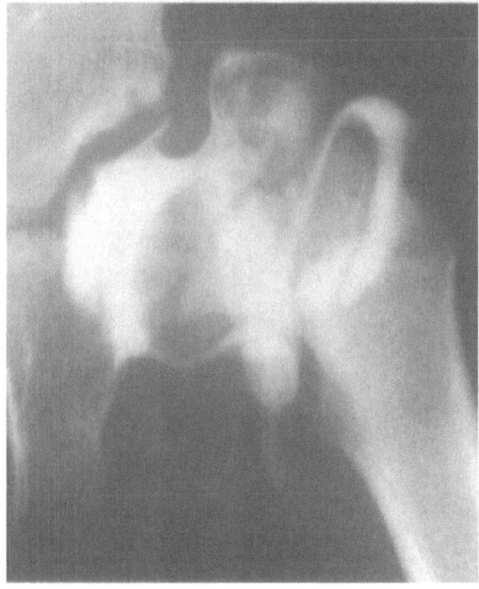

C85.2

Case 85.   Answers:

1. The capital femoral epiphysis is flattened, small and fragmented and incompletely covered by the poorly formed acetabular roof. The femoral neck is short and broad. The arthrogram shows that part of the capital femoral epiphysis is within and part without the irregular acetabulum (changes of old septic arthritis).

2. The computed tomogram (C85.3) shows the relationship of the capital femoral epiphysis and femoral neck to the acetabulum in the transverse plane. There is anteversion of the femoral neck here.

3. Synovitis; septic arthritis; Perthes' disease; chronic osteomyelitis; stress fracture; osteoid osteoma; mono-articular rheumatoid arthritis; slipped capital femoral epiphysis (C85.4).

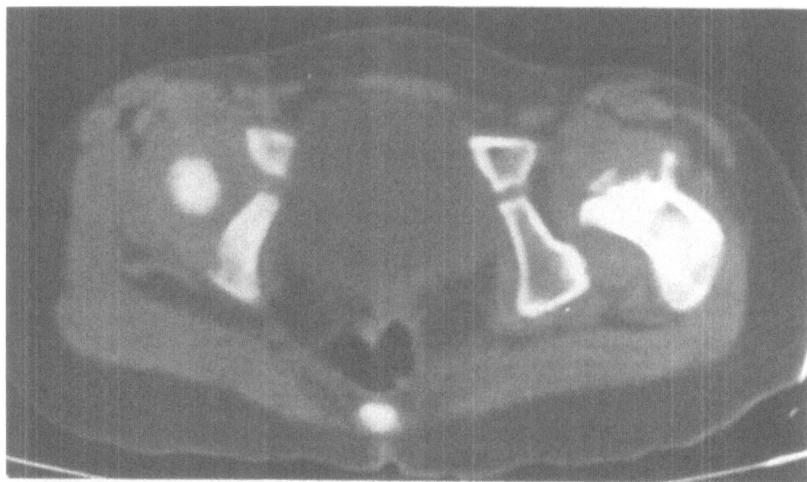

C85.3

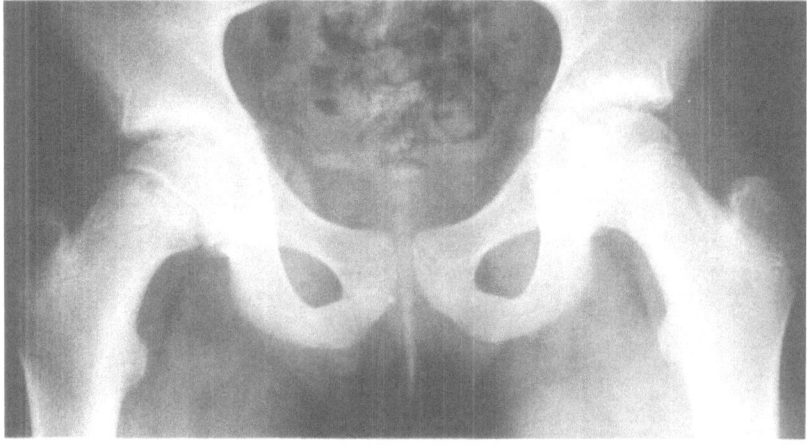

C85.4

Case 86.   This 1-month-old neonate was unwell and irritable on handling.

Questions:

1. Describe the abnormalities of the right lower limb (C86.1).
2. Describe the abnormalities of the left lower limb.
3. What is the diagnosis on the right?
4. What is the diagnosis on the left?
5. What is the likely cause?

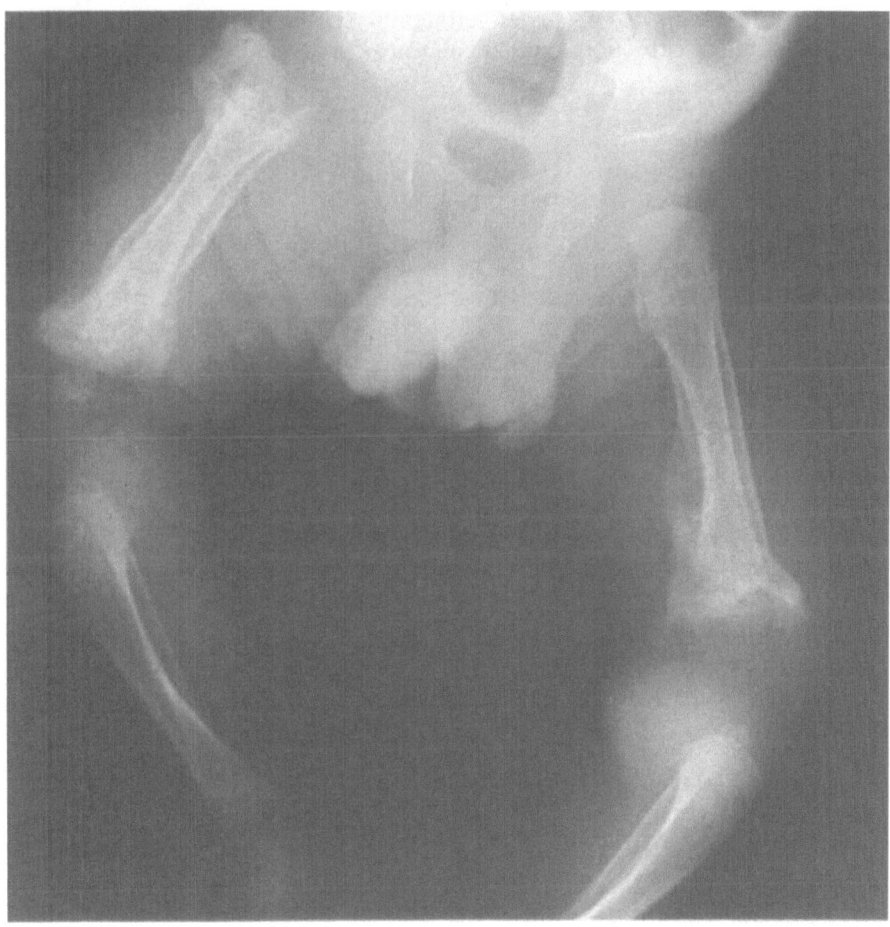

C86.1

Case 86. Answers:

1. Dislocated right hip and extensive new bone formation involving the whole femur.
2. Destruction of the lower femoral epiphysis, irregularity of the metaphysis and extensive new bone formation along the femoral shaft.
3. A septic arthritis of the hip with osteomyelitis.
4. A septic arthritis of the knee with osteomyelitis.
5. Septicaemia due to *Staphylococcus aureus*.

Case 86. Comments:

C86.2 and C86.3 show long-term results. The right hip remains dislocated with destruction of the capital femoral epiphysis and femoral neck (unlike congenital dislocation of the hip). The lower left femur shows a "chevron" deformity caused by partial destruction and irregular growth at the epiphyseal plate.

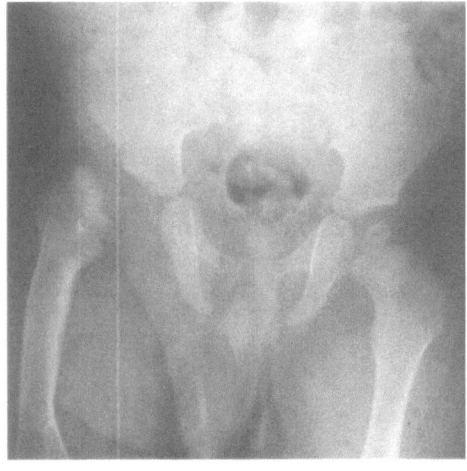

C86.2

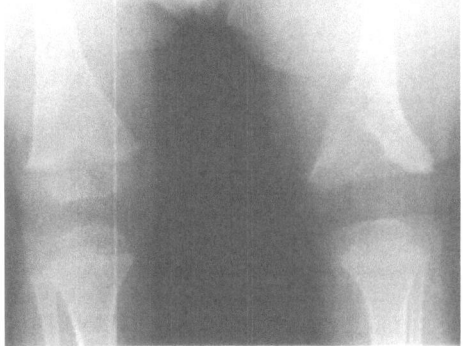

C86.3

Case 87. This 2-month-old infant presented with irritability on being handled and painful swelling of both forearms and legs and of the lower jaw.

Questions:

1. Describe the changes in the forearms (C87.1; C87.2).
2. What is the diagnosis?
3. What is the differential diagnosis?
4. What long-term complications of this condition may result?

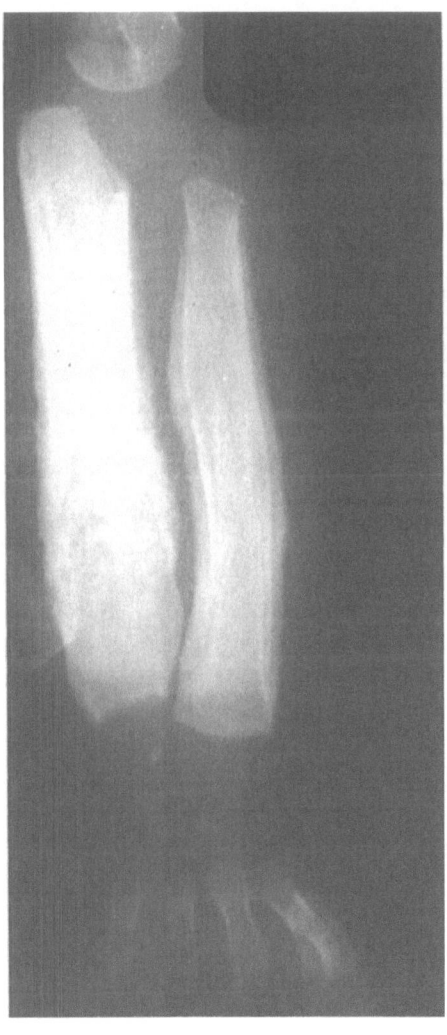

C87.1

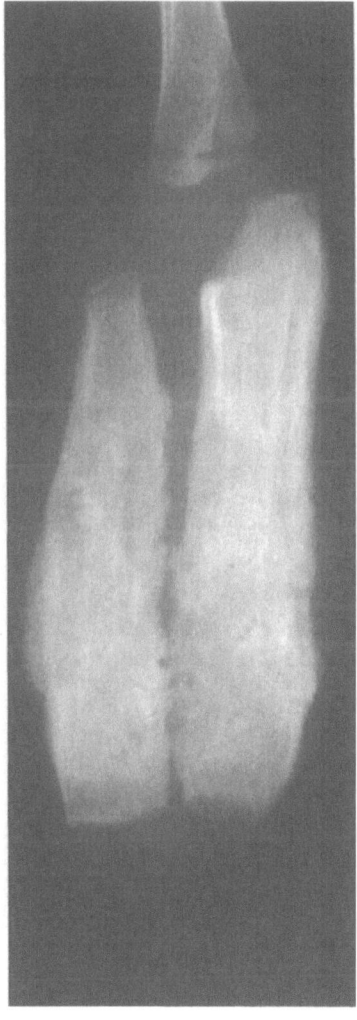

C87.2

173

Case 87. Answers:

1. Extensive periosteal reactions involving diaphyses and distal metaphyses.

2. Caffey's disease (idiopathic cortical hyperostosis).

3. a) Multifocal osteomyelitis.
   b) Leukaemic infiltration (not under 6 months of age).
   c) Neuroblastoma (metastatic) usually with some patchy lysis.
   d) Congenital syphilis.
   e) Subperiosteal bleeding (rickets, scurvy, trauma), but in these conditions the mandible is rarely affected and the changes are rarely symmetrical.

4. Cross-fusion of adjacent bones with potential respiratory embarrassment if rib fusion occurs.

Case 88.   This infant presented with failure to thrive and pain on being handled.

Questions:

1. Describe the changes at the metaphysis of the lower femur (C88.1).
2. Describe the appearances of the epiphyses.
3. What is the diagnosis?

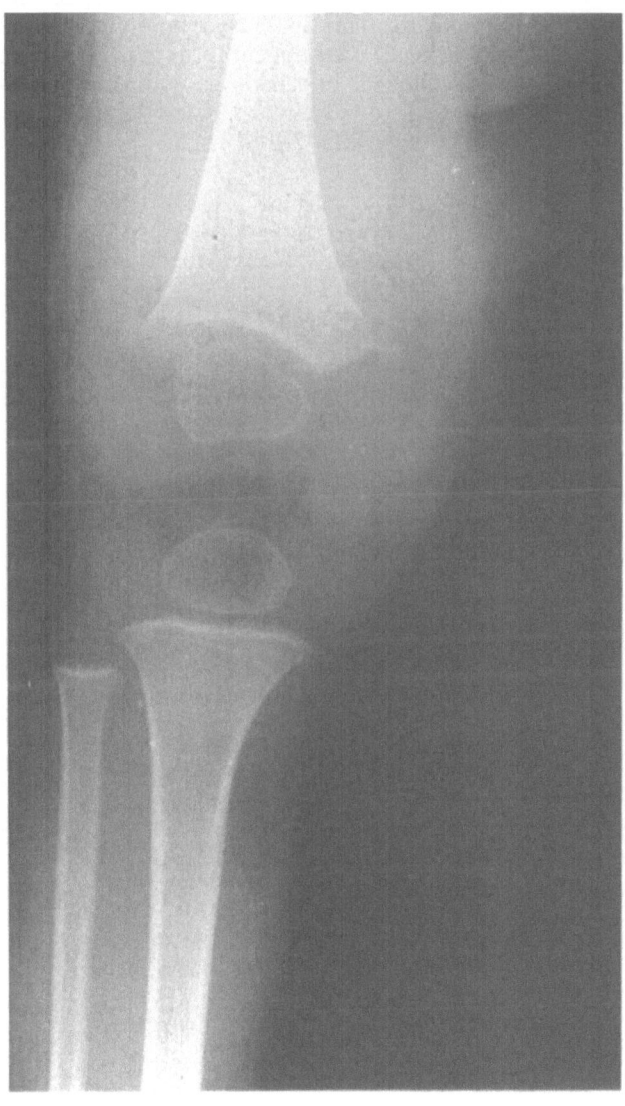

C88.1

Case 88. Answers:

1. There are metaphyseal fractures of the lower femoral metaphysis giving rise to the "pelkan spur" appearance.
2. They have a pencil-thin cortical outline; the "ring sign" of Wimberger.
3. Scurvy.

Case 88. Comments:

Similar metaphyseal fractures may be seen in non-accidental injury and in Menkes' kinky hair syndrome. C88.2 demonstrates extensive new-bone formation around the lower femoral metaphysis. This is caused by subperiosteal bleeding resulting from the effects of scurvy. Similar appearances may be seen in any bleeding disorder. C88.3 illustrates changes in a neonate with thrombocytopoenia.

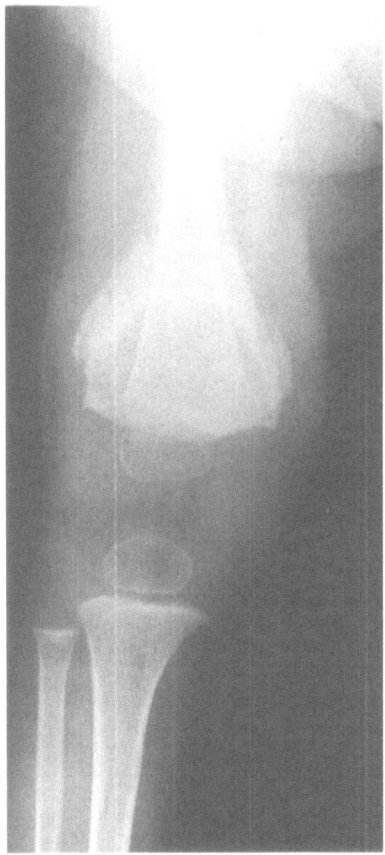

C88.2

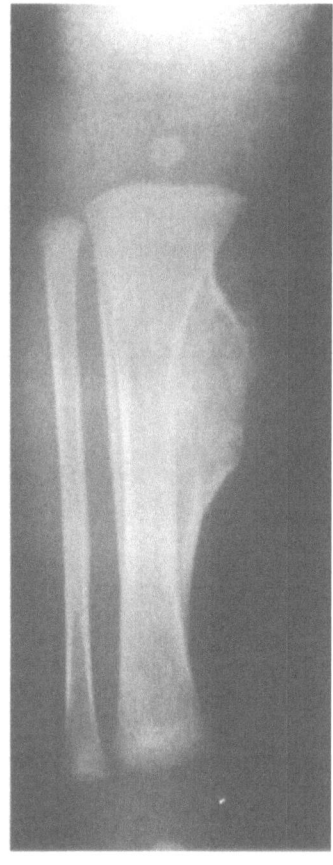

C88.3

Case 89. A 2-month-old infant presented with a swollen left leg and with a history of having rolled off the bed.

Questions:

1. Describe the changes at the distal tibial metaphysis (C89.1).
2. What other investigation would you recommend and why?

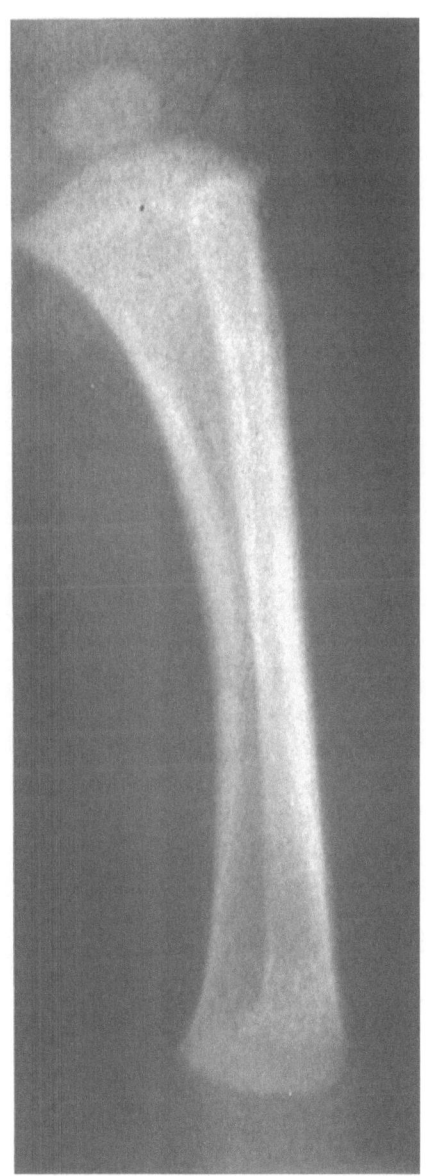

C89.1

Case 89. Answers:

1. There is an entire rim of metaphysis separated from the shaft. This a "bucket-handle" fracture and is caused by a twisting and pulling action (not by accidental trauma). It is a feature of non-accidental injury.

2. A full skeletal survey because of the type of bony injury and the vague history.

Case 89. Comments:

The appearances of the tibia and fibula 2 weeks later are shown (C89.2) with extensive periosteal new bone along the diaphysis and with metaphyseal fractures now of the proximal metaphyses. Similar metaphyseal fractures are a feature of scurvy and of Menkes' kinky hair syndrome (C89.3) in which there is disordered copper metabolism and progressive neurological degeneration.

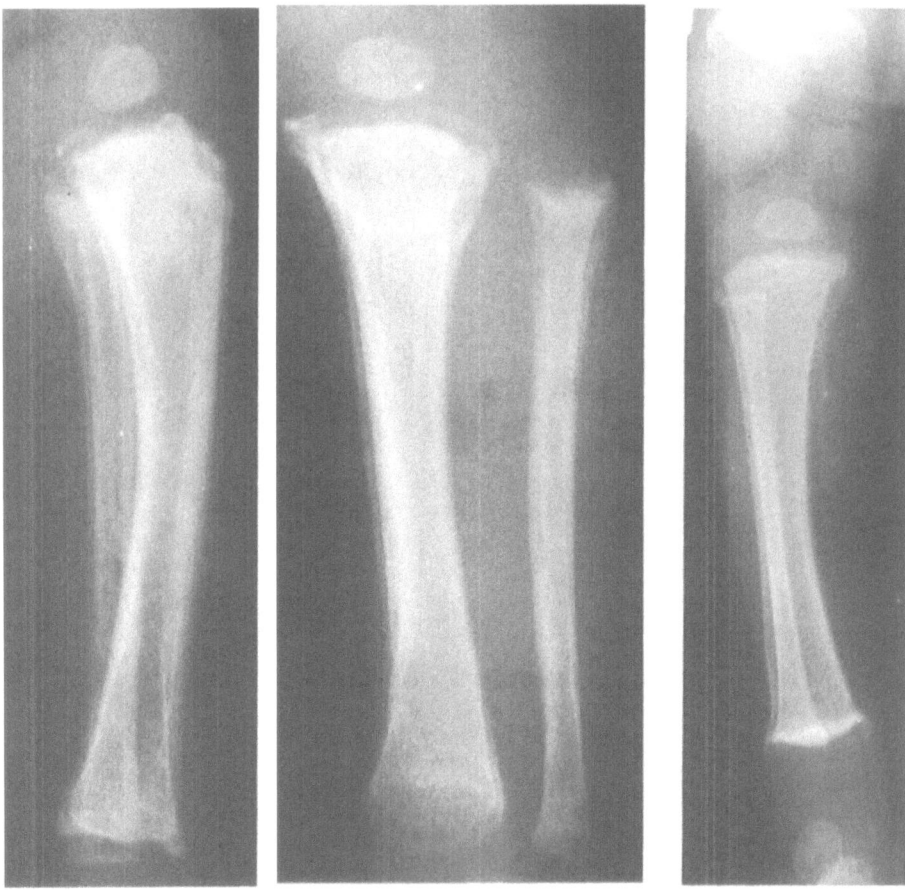

C89.2   C89.3

Case 90. This 12-year-old presented with pain of several weeks' duration in his right leg.

Questions:

1. Describe the findings on these AP (C90.1) and lateral (C90.2) views of his left tibia and fibula.
2. What is the differential diagnosis?
3. Name two other investigations which may be helpful.
4. What further history would you try to elicit?

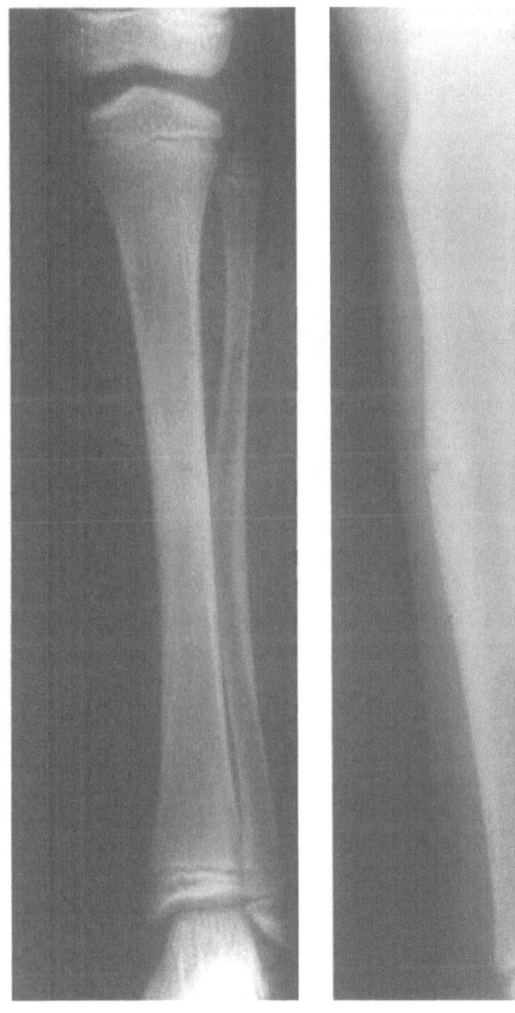

C90.1   C90.2

179

Case 90. Answers:

1. On the lateral view there is marked thickening of the tibia due to organised periosteal new bone anteriorly. A localised radiolucent area is present where the cortex is most thick.

2. a) Osteoid osteoma.
   b) Stress fracture (final diagnosis).

3. a) Tomography (may demonstrate the dense central nidus of an osteoid osteoma).
   b) Radionuclide bone scan (very localised and marked increased uptake of isotope at the site of the osteoid osteoma nidus). In the presence of a stress fracture there is increased uptake in the early blood-pool phase.

4. Osteoid osteoma is characteristically relieved by aspirin. Stress fractures in this position are caused by running and jumping and may be seen in ballet dancers.

Case 91.   This neonate has shortening and bowing of the right leg.

Questions:

1. Describe the bony changes (C91.1).
2. What is the differential diagnosis?

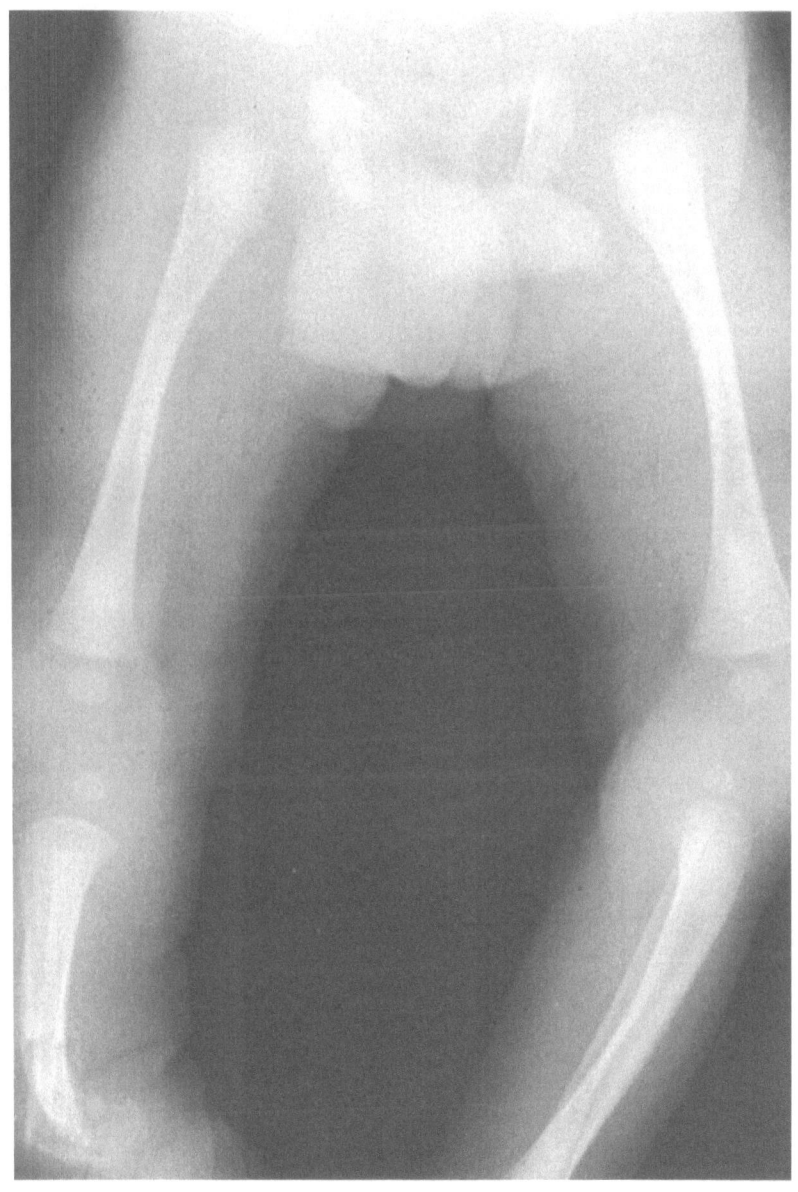

C91.1

Case 91. Answers:

1. There is forward angulation of the lower tibia and fibula (a pseudoarthrosis), with radiolucent areas and some expansion.

2. Neurofibromatosis (final diagnosis); fibrous dysplasia (monostotic) (C91.2).

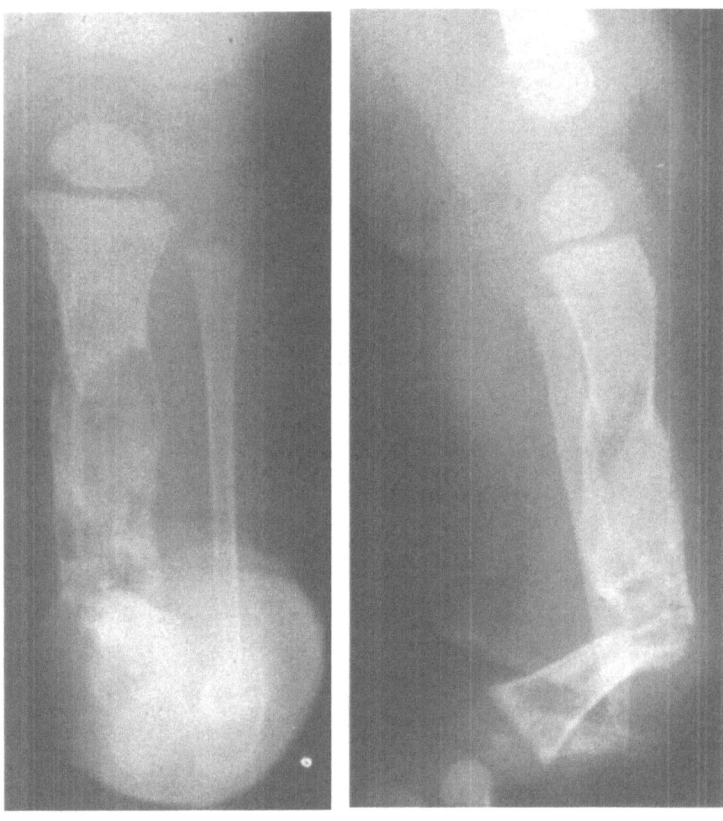

C91.2

Case 92. **This neonate was found to have clicking hips when examined by the paediatrician.**

Questions:

1. Describe the abnormalities on the radiograph of the pelvis with the hips in the neutral position (C92.1).

2. What is the diagnosis?

3. How is the condition managed (a) initially and (b) in later childhood?

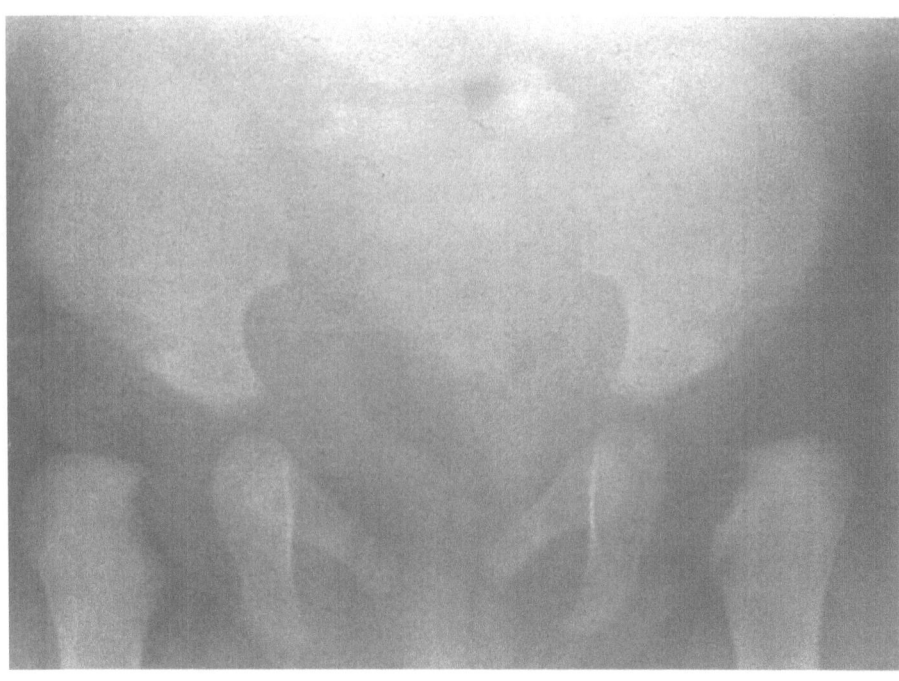

C92.1

Case 92. Answers:

1. The acetabular roofs are shallow and slope steeply. The femoral necks are in valgus and the capital femoral epiphyses, as yet unossified, but lying above the femoral metaphyses, lie outside the lateral acetabular angles.

2. Congenital dislocation of the hips.

3. a) Abduction harness/splint for several months.
   b) Corrective osteotomy—either femoral shaft or iliac "shelf" procedure.

Case 92. Comments:

C92.2 illustrates dislocation of the left hip secondary to old septic arthritis. Without the continuing stimulus of weight bearing, the acetabulum fails to develop normally. A pseudoacetabulum has formed. The capital femoral epiphysis is virtually destroyed and the upper femoral metaphysis is irregular.

In congenitally dislocated hips the capital femoral epiphyses ossify late (normally visible at 6 months). Manipulation may result in avascular necrosis.

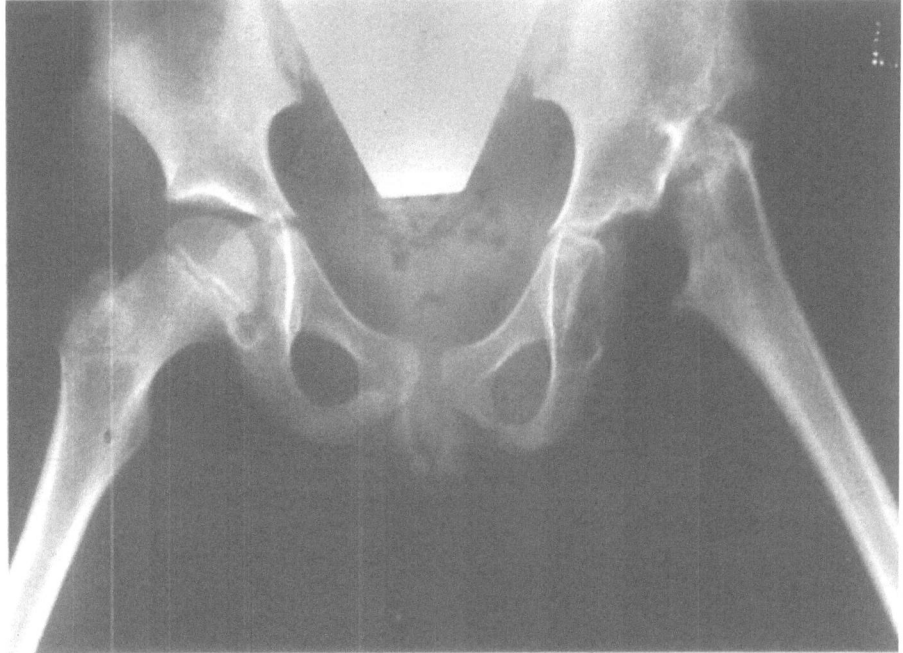

C92.2

Case 93. This 6-month-old infant presented with gross unilateral soft tissue abnormalities.

Questions:

1. Describe the bony abnormalities (C93.1).
2. What is the differential diagnosis?
3. What long-term follow-up would you recommend?

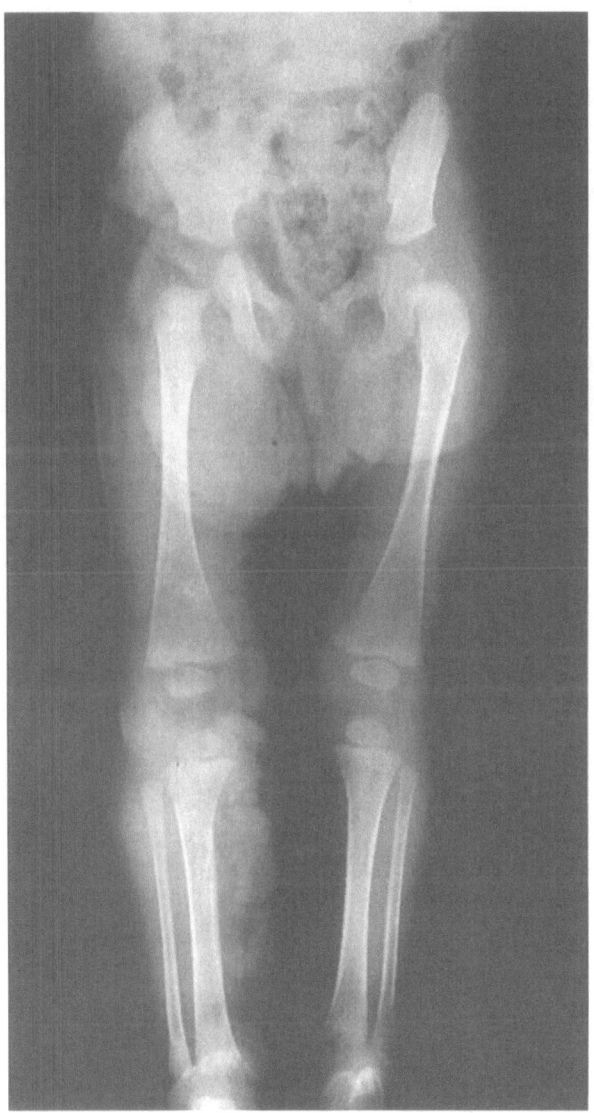

C93.1

Case 93. Answers:

1. Right-sided hemihypertrophy; increased bone length and advanced bone maturation compared with the left.

2. Haemangioma; Klippel-Trenaunay syndrome (venous); lymphangiomatosis; neurofibromatosis.

3. Three- to six-monthly abdominal ultrasound because of the risk of abdominal malignancy in hemihypertrophy.

Case 93. Comments:

Conditions associated with hemihypertrophy:

Tumours—Wilms', neuroblastoma, hepatoblastoma, adrenal carcinoma or adenoma.

Vascular—haemangioma, Klippel-Trenaunay syndrome. Lymphangiomatosis.

Renal—medullary sponge kidney, Wilms' tumour, renal hypertrophy, Beckwith-Wiedemann syndrome, hypospadias/cryptorchidism.

Neurocutaneous syndromes—neurofibromatosis, von-Hippel-Lindau disease, Ehlers-Danlos syndrome.

Pyloric stenosis.

Russell-Silver dwarf syndrome.

Case 94. **This 8-year-old girl has pain in her back.**

Questions:

1. Describe the skeletal abnormalities on the lateral thoraco-lumbar radiograph (C94.1).
2. List the possible causes of this appearance.

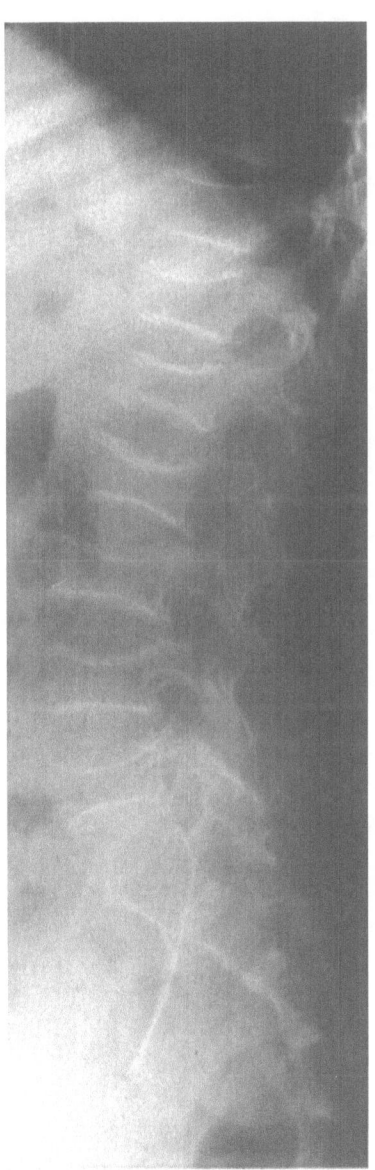

C94.1

187

Case 94. Answers:

1. There is generalised biconcave flattening of the vertebral bodies associated with marked osteoporosis (sometimes called the "cod-fish" appearance, referring to the shape of the intervertebral spaces).

2. Osteogenesis Imperfecta (final diagnosis); idiopathic juvenile osteoporosis; hepatoblastoma when associated with osteoporosis; prolonged steroid therapy; Cushing's syndrome; thyrotoxicosis; leukaemia; metastatic neuroblastoma; homocystinuria; Gaucher's disease.

Case 94. Comments:

This boy presented with pathological metaphyseal fractures (C94.2). He was found to have an hepatoblastoma. C94.3 illustrates the generalised vertebral collapse. Following resection of the hepatoblastoma the osteoporosis improved and vertebral body height increased.

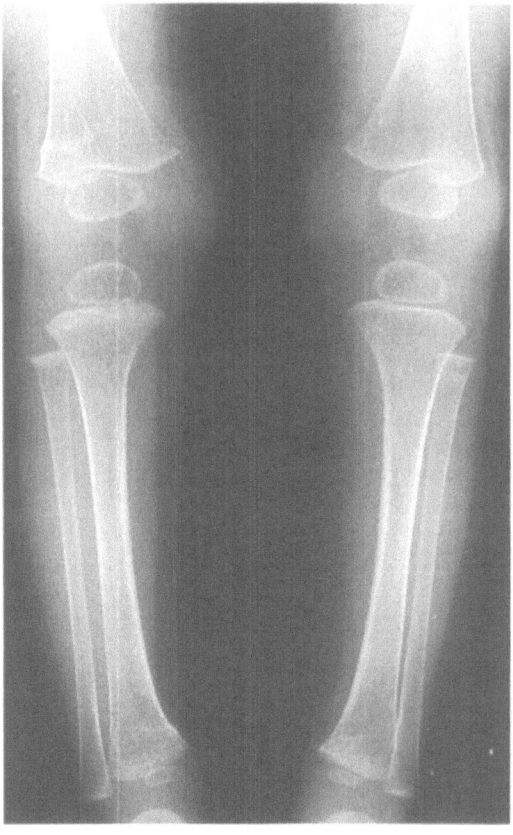

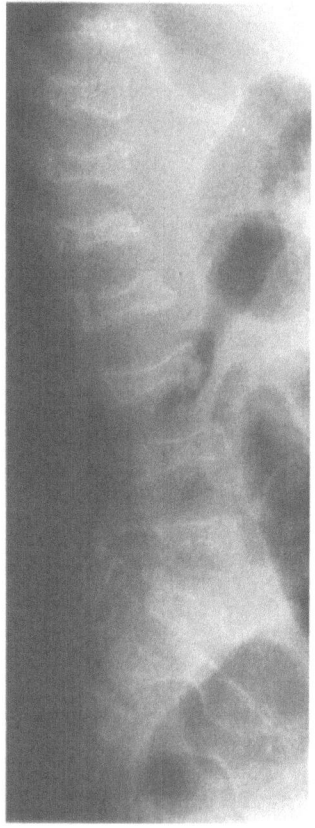

C94.2   C94.3

Case 95.   This 2-year-old girl is mentally retarded due to a neonatal intracerebral bleed. She has bilaterally symmetrical forearm deformities.

Questions:

1. What are the radiological abnormalities of the left forearm (C95.1)?
2. What is the diagnosis?

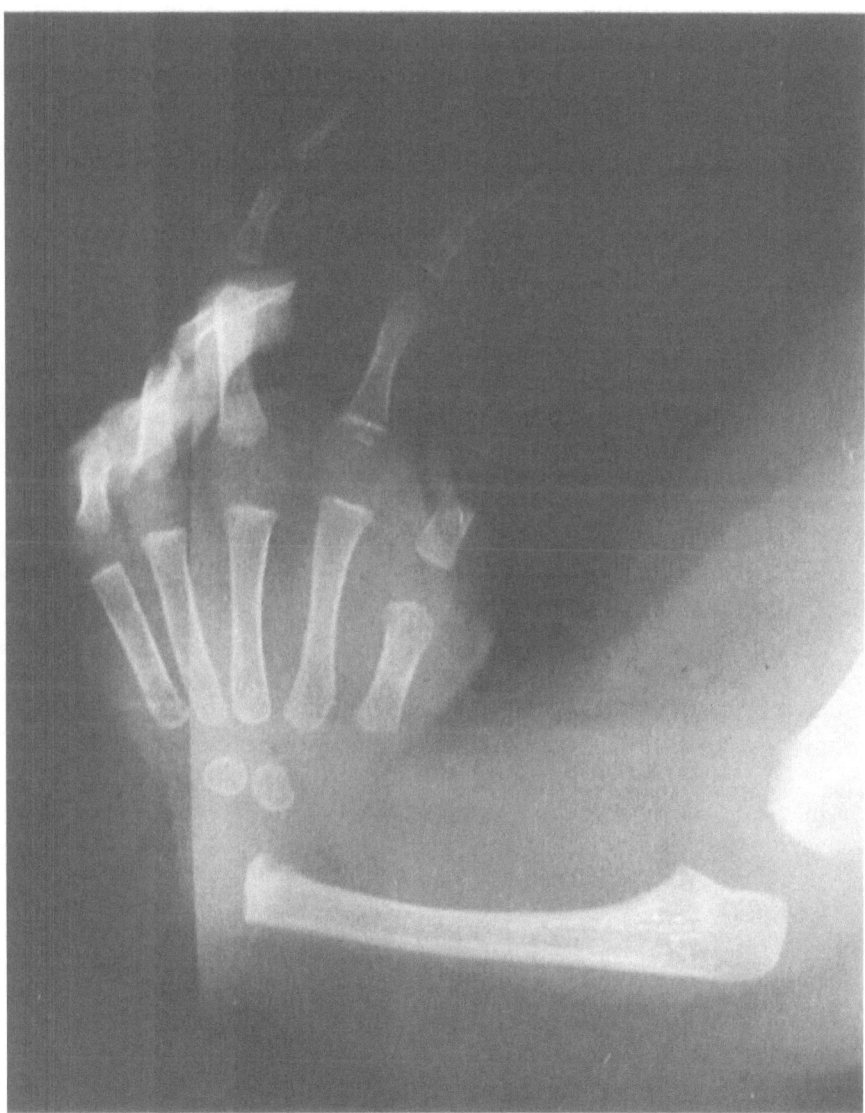

C95.1

Case 95. Answers:

1. Absence of the radius, but with normal digits. Radial deviation at the wrist.
2. TAR (thrombocytopoenia absent radius) syndrome.

Case 95. Comments:

In this condition the thumb is characteristically normal. Most other radial hypoplasia/absence defects affect the thumb. Causes of bilateral radial ray hypoplasia include: TAR; Fanconi's anaemia; VATER association; Holt-Oram syndrome. C95.2 shows absent thumb and a small os centrale at the bases of the capitate and hamate and C95.3 shows fusion of proximal and distal carpal bones and radial hypoplasia both in a patient with the Holt-Oram syndrome.

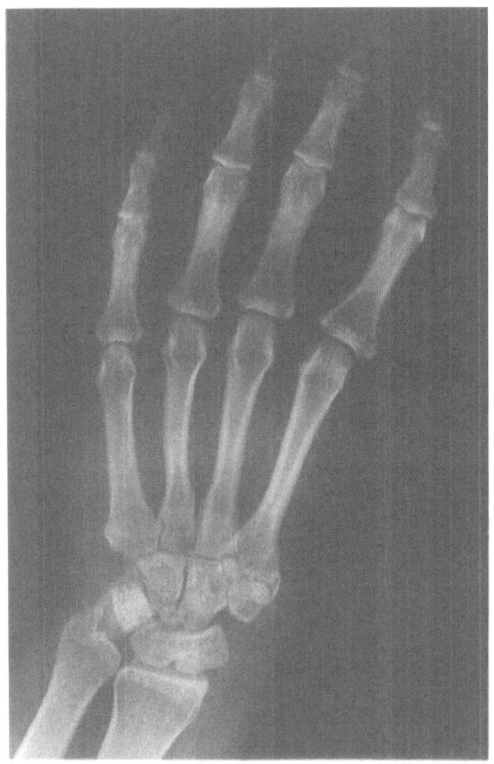

C95.2

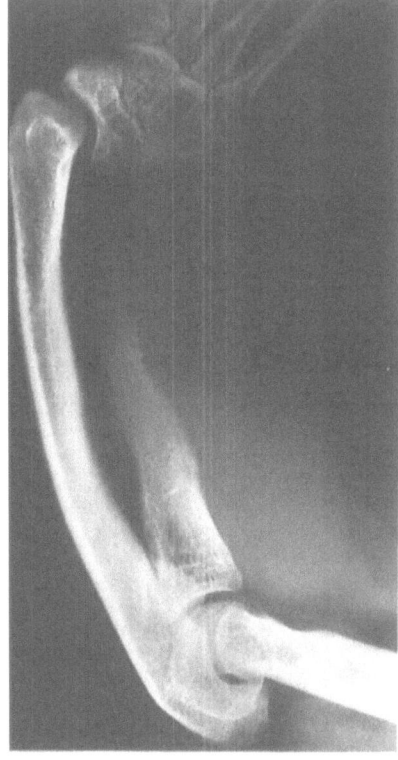

C95.3

Case 96. This 3-year-old boy presented with bilateral congenital forearm deformities and a urinary tract infection. He is now aged 7 and has become anaemic.

Questions:

1. Describe the bony abnormalities (C96.1).
2. What is the name used to describe this deformity?
3. What is the diagnosis?
4. Is the urinary tract infection significant and why?

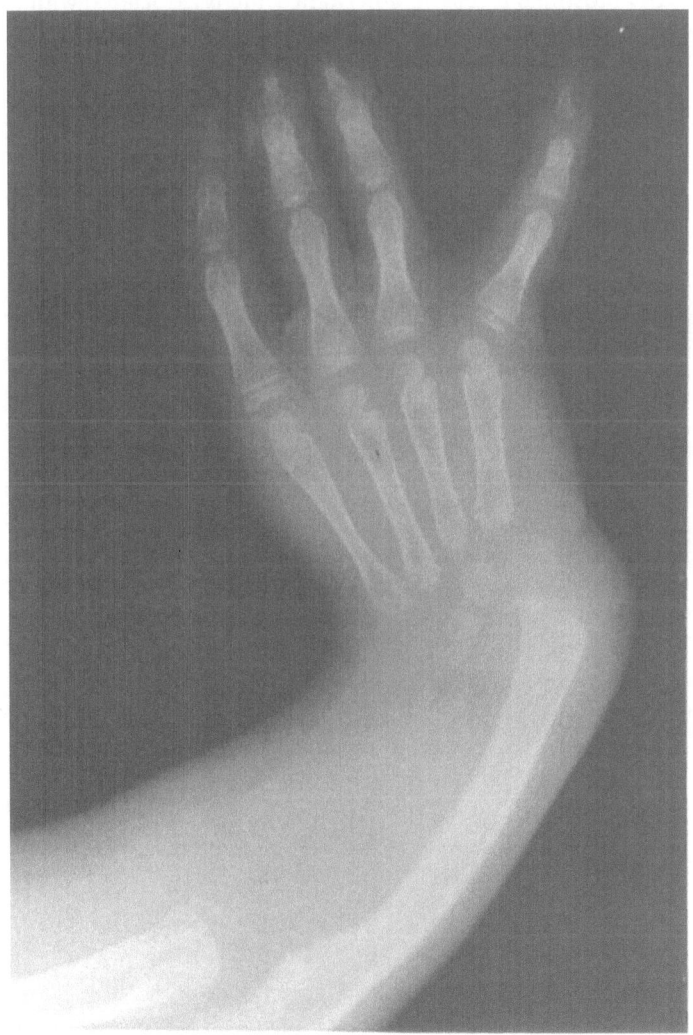

C96.1

Case 96. Answers:

1. Absent radius and thumb with radial deviation of the hand and a bowed ulna.
2. Radial club hand.
3. Fanconi's anaemia.
4. Yes. Congenital renal abnormalities, e.g. duplex, pelvic, crossed-fused ectopia, are associated with Fanconi's anaemia and all predispose to urinary tract infections.

Case 96. Comments:

This patient's IVU tomogram (C96.2) demonstrates bilateral pelvic kidneys. Fanconi's anaemia is of autosomal recessive inheritance and is associated with an increased incidence of malignancies.

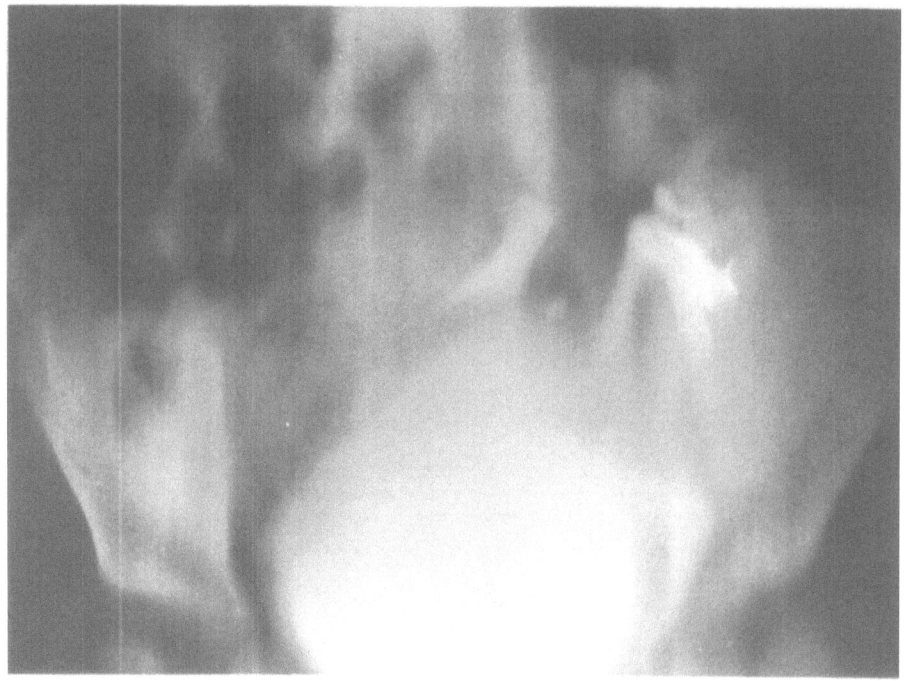

C96.2

Case 97.   This 18-month-old girl had oesophageal atresia repaired as a neonate.

Questions:

1. Describe the abnormality (C97.1).
2. What other congenital abnormalities could she have had?

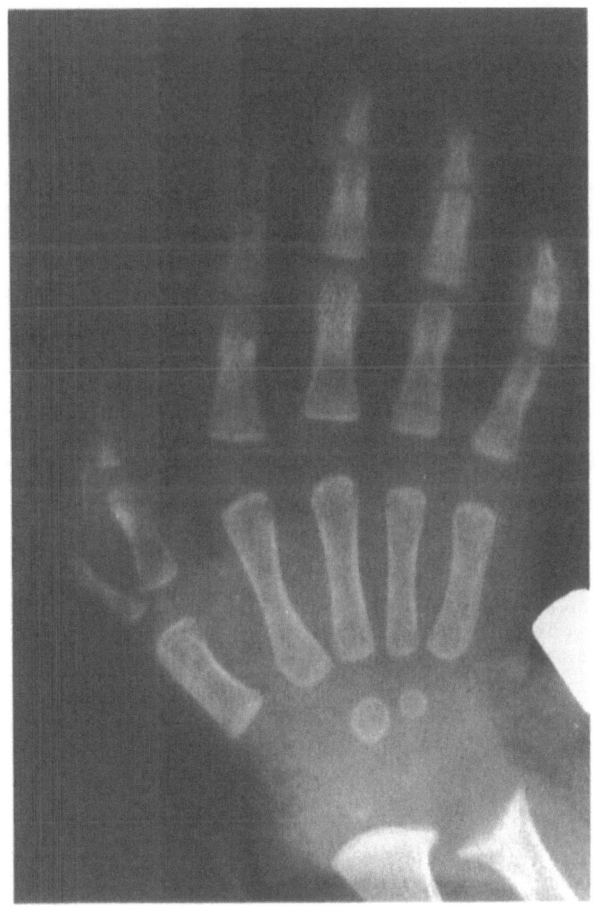

C97.1

Case 97. Answers:

1. Pre-axial polydactyly with duplication of the thumb.
2. V, vascular, vertebral
   A, anorectal atresia
   R, renal abnormalities (C97.2).
   These are all part of the VATER association.

Case 97. Comments:

This type of duplication of the thumb is the commonest form of radial ray abnormality in the VATER association. Other conditions associated with pre-axial (thumb) polydactyly include: absent tibia; Fanconi's anaemia; Oro-facio-digital syndrome; Holt-Oram syndrome; Carpenter's acrocephalopolysyndactyly.

C97.2 shows right-sided colostomy for anorectal atresia, solitary left kidney and six lumbar vertebrae. C97.3 (renogram) confirms the presence of a solitary left kidney.

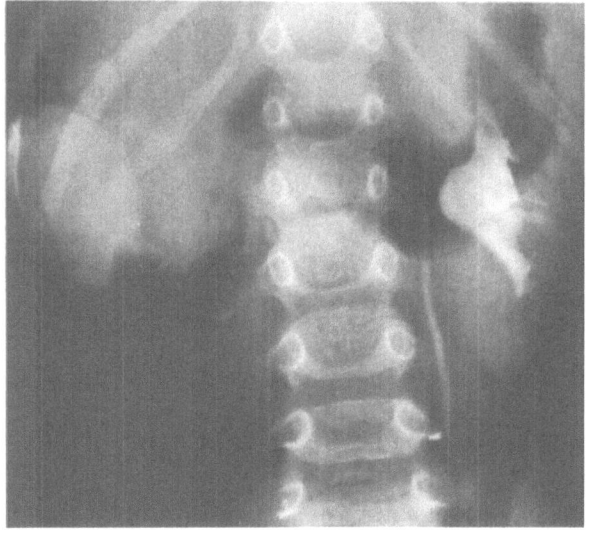

C97.2

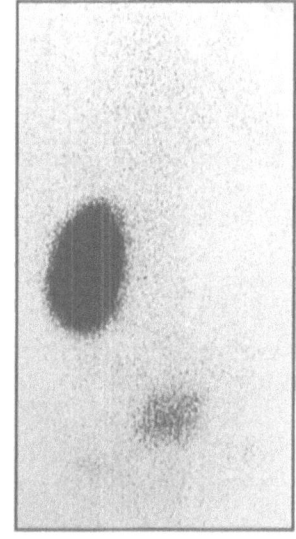

C97.3

Case 98.   This 6-year-old girl with a chronic disorder presented with progressive weakness of her legs.

Questions:

1. a) Describe the shape of the skull vault (C98.1).
    b) Name the abnormalities seen in the lambdoid sutures.
    c) Describe two abnormalities of the skull base.

2. What is the diagnosis of this chronic disorder?

3. Why does she have leg weakness?

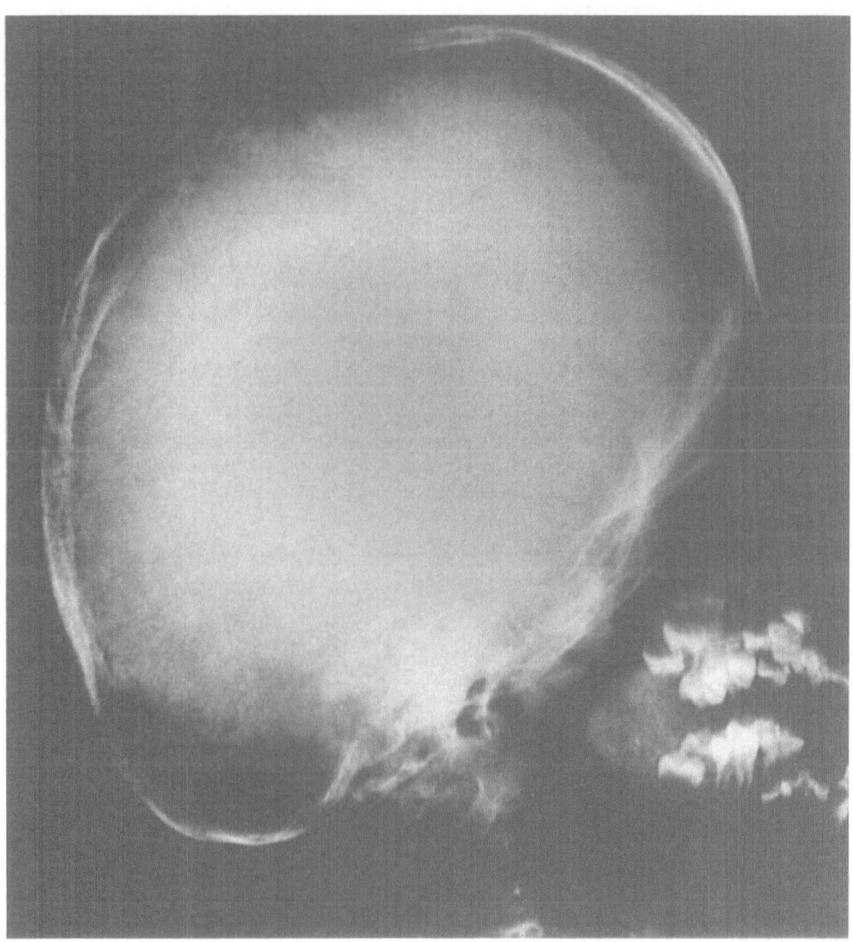

C98.1

Case 98. Answers:

1. a) Brachycephaly.
   b) Wormian bones.
   c) Platybasia (basilar invagination) and elongated pituitary fossa.
2. Osteogenesis imperfecta.
3. Paraplegia due to progressive basilar invagination.

Case 98. Comments:

Other radiological features of osteogenesis imperfecta include: osteoporosis; multiple fractures; exuberant callus formation; occasional pseudarthrosis; deformity—limbs and spine; osteosarcoma—rare complication.

Other rare conditions in which there is osteoporosis with fracturing and Wormian bones include Menke's kinky hair syndrome, Hajdu-Cheyney syndrome and cutis laxa.

Case 99. This 4-year-old boy has coarse facies and corneal opacities.

Questions:

Describe the appearances of:
1. The skull (C99.1).

2. The spine (C99.2).

3. The chest (C99.3).

4. The hand (C99.4).

5. What is the diagnosis?

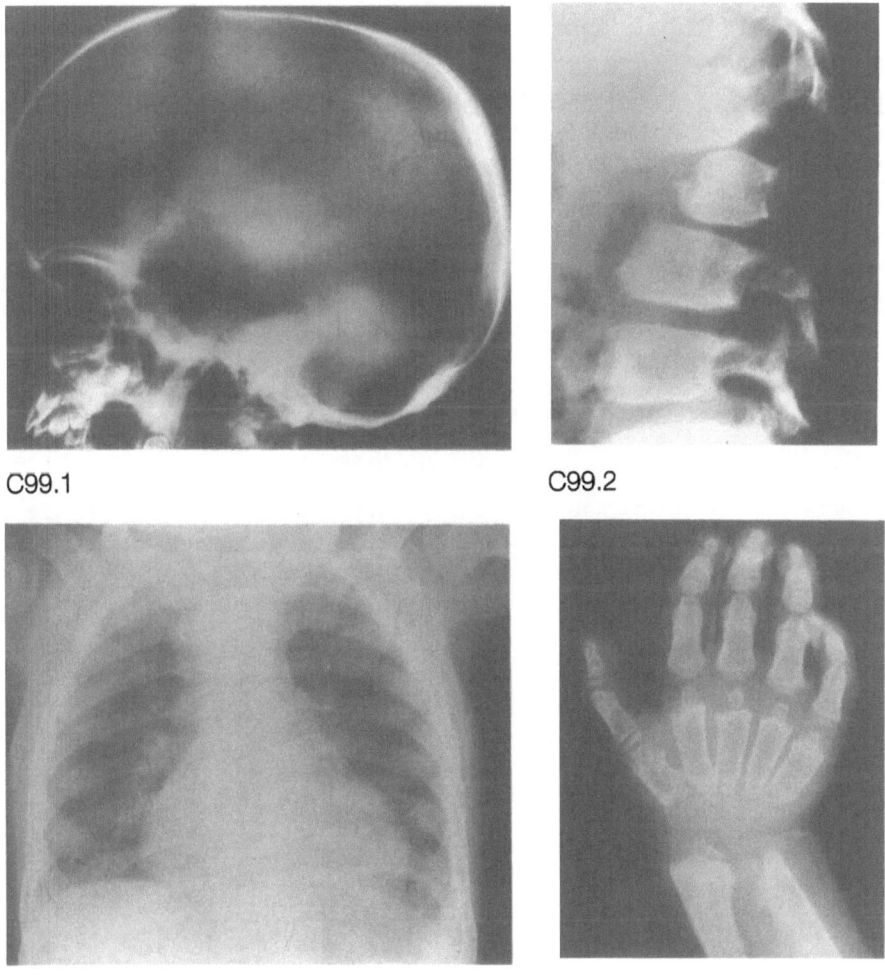

C99.1

C99.2

C99.3

C99.4

Case 99. Answers:

1. Large vault; splayed sutures indicating raised intracranial pressure; overall "ground-glass" opacity; elongated, J-shaped sella; pointed condylar processes of the mandible.

2. Oval configuration with posterior scalloping; inferior hooks L2 and L3; hypoplasia of L2 with a kyphos.

3. Large heart; broad ribs.

4. Short sloping distal ulna; proximal pointing of second to fifth metacarpals; "bullet" shaped phalanges (broader at their bases than distally).

5. One of the mucopolysaccharidoses. It is difficult radiologically to differentiate between type I-H (Hurler), type II (Hunter) and type VI (Maroteaux-Lamy).

Case 99. Comments:

The figures below (C99.5; C99.6) illustrate the typical spine changes in a child with mucopolysaccharidosis type IV (Morquio disease). There is platyspondyly with anterior "tonguing" and an absent odontoid peg with instability.

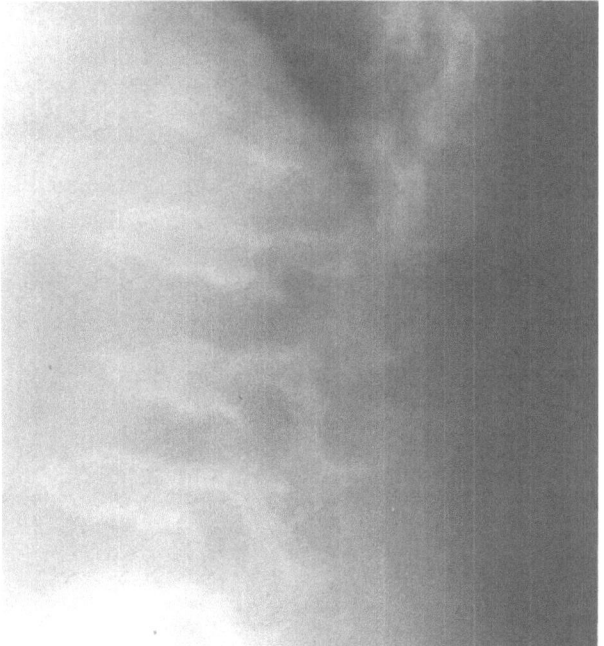

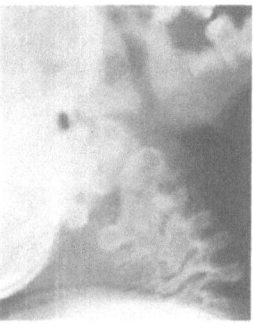

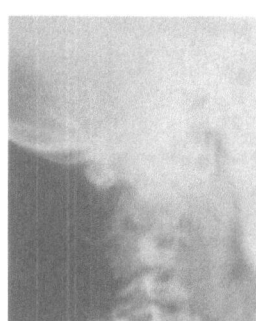

C99.5   C99.6

Case 100. These are AP (C.100.1) and lateral (C100.2) radiographs of a still-born, short limbed neonate.

Questions:

1. Describe the appearances of the long bones.
2. Describe the spinal appearances.
3. What is the descriptive name given to the femora?
4. What is the diagnosis?
5. Name two other conditions which are still-born with short limbs?

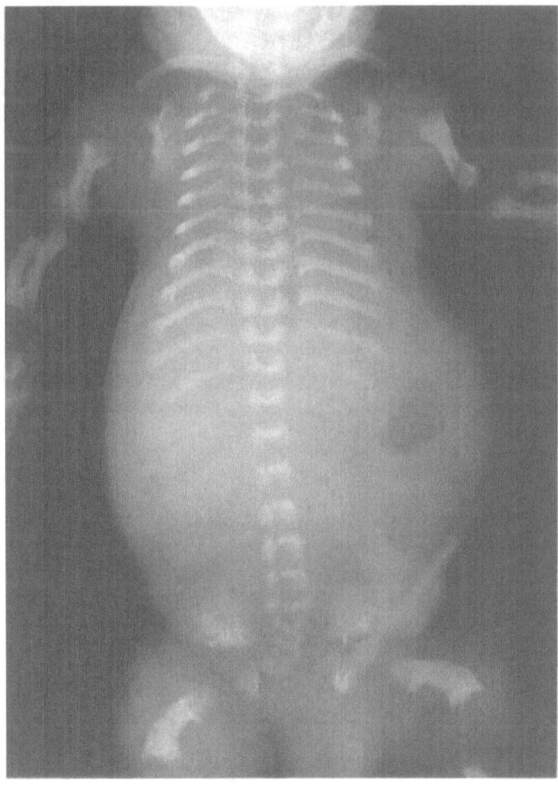

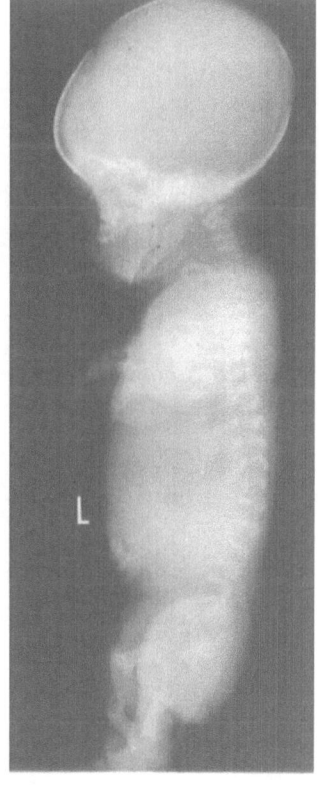

C100.1   C100.2

Case 100.   Answers:

1. All are short with metaphyseal irregularity/cupping and there is bowing of the femoral shafts.
2. There is platyspondyly. On the AP view the vertebral bodies have an "H" configuration.
3. "Telephone-handle" deformity.
4. Thanatophoric dysplasia.
5. Achondrogenesis (C100.3).
   Short-ribbed-polydactyly syndromes.

Case 100.   Comments:

Achondrogenesis demonstrates the most severe form of long bone shortening. In addition there is absent ossification of part of the spine and poor vault ossification. Other potentially lethal conditions, with limb shortening and poorly ossified vault bones include hypophosphatasia and osteogenesis imperfecta.

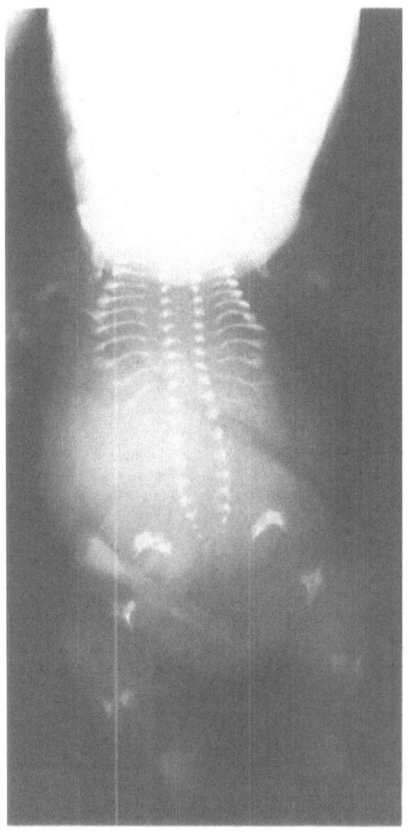

C100.3

Subject Index